THE COMPLETE GUIDE

TO THE STREET DRUG GAME

THE COMPLETE GUIDE TO THE STREET DRUG GAME

By Scott R. French

lyle stuart inc.

Secaucus, N. J. 07094

First printing, April 1976
Second printing, August 1976

Queries regarding rights and permissions
should be addressed to:
Lyle Stuart, Inc.
120 Enterprise Avenue
Secaucus, N. J. 07094

Manufactured in the United States of America

Published simultaneously in Canada by
George J. McLeod Limited, Toronto, Ontario

ISBN 0-8184-0208-3—*hardcover*
ISBN 0-8184-0237-7—*paperbound*

I would like to dedicate this book to my wife, Margaret, who spent many late hours editing and typesetting, and without whose help there would be no book. . .

TABLE OF CONTENTS

ACKNOWLEDGEMENTS

Although this book was "written" by me, many people, including a number of freaks, doctors, chemists, and even a narc or two helped with the research and material. I would like to express my appreciation to all who contributed a bit of themselves.

Art by: Alfred Klostermann
Lance Lough

The author and publishers of this book do not wish to encourage anyone to take drugs of any nature. The information contained herein is for purposes of information ONLY, and we can bear no responsibility for the utilization of any procedures listed.

Much of this book is written in a colloquial language such as that employed by winos, freaks, and drug users. If you are a reviewer, librarian, or member of a law enforcement agency and do not understand parts of it, drop me a line in care of the publishers and I will do what I can to help. . .

THE COMPLETE GUIDE

TO THE STREET DRUG GAME

NARCS AND ROBBERS

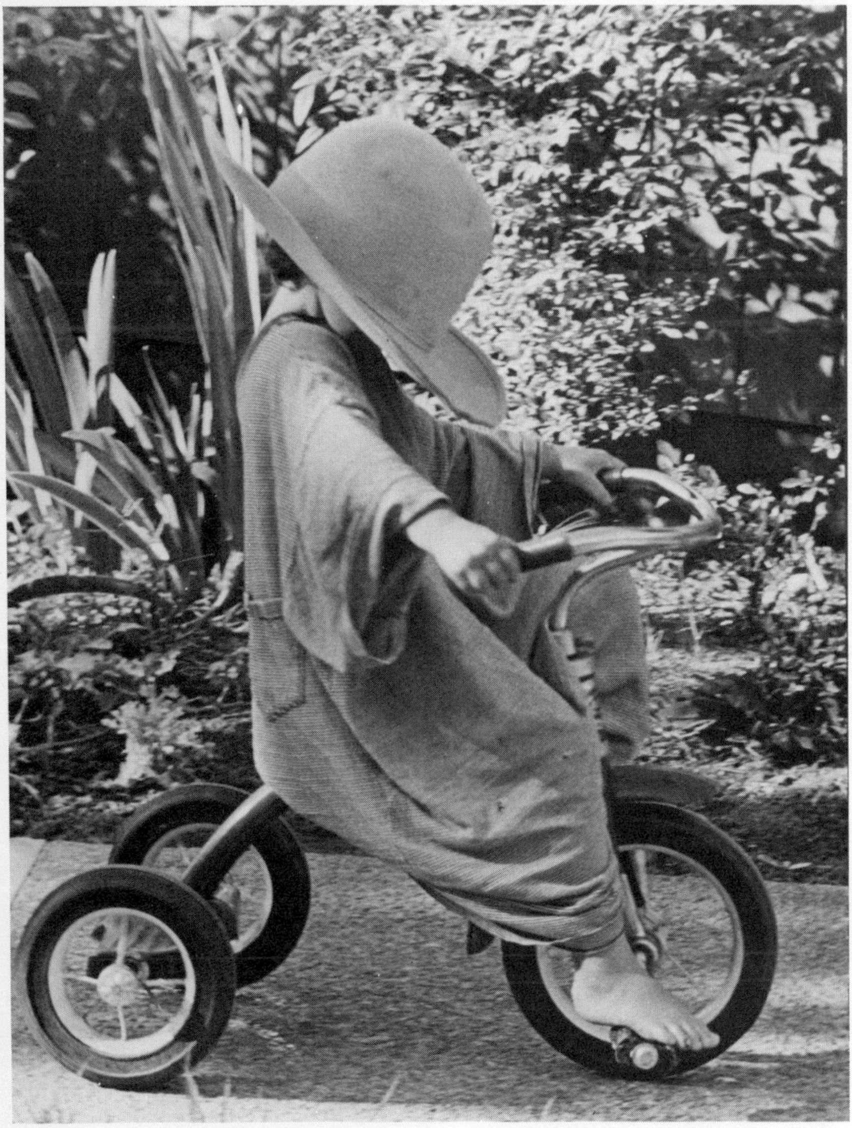

NARCS AND ROBBERS

The term "narc" is an ambiguous, viable term applied with equal ferocity to local police, state investigators, The Drug Enforcement Administration and, on occasion, to informers, suspected informers, and just enemies.

LOCALS

Local narcs are a bit different than their federal counterparts. The local may not have wanted the drug detail or he may really dig the idea, but he knows his effectiveness is limited to the time he can operate without undue recognition. In some areas this may be as little as three to six months, seldom longer than a couple of years.

If he wants promotions, it means a lot of busts on the record, so the local is more likely to bust small-time users, use drugs himself (many locals will smoke grass, or use coke – few will shoot or use heavy psychedelics) and generally bust weaker cases. He probably isn't getting paid as much as his federal counterparts, may not have the same education or standards, and will be more likely to be a real longhair, grubby type.

Due to his limited operation period and his smaller pay scale (although not small by any means – how many college graduates can get $800 to $1,000 right out of school, as one can in the L.A.P.D.?), the local is much more likely to have a side trip or two – notably rip-offs and occasionally dealing.

Many police departments have given narcotics the top priority, and have increased their narcotic staff by as much as several hundred per cent. This, ludicrously, is increased when you realize judges and parole officers, always on the lookout to please the public, tend to concentrate heavily on "vogue" crimes. This means we often have the grass smoker or "pusher" getting big time while the assault or armed robber gets a slap in the face and a taste of county time.

In some metropolitan areas, such as New York and San Francisco, the chances of getting ripped off, as well as busted, when turned by a local agent are much greater than 50/50. The average seems to be to take any cash found in the defendant's possession, house, or where he is busted and report a small amount (seems to run about $500 reported for every $2,000 – $5,000 grabbed), take stereos and camera equipment, anything which looks vaguely illegal or might be used as a "weapon" and nicer clothes, (if near the agent's size).

Many cops look forward to the drug detail, again, especially in larger cities, as sort of a pre-retirement plan. They reason "you know where it came from," and "he'd just spend it on some fancy lawyer to try and beat it, and he is guilty," so why turn it over to the courts and possibly back to the defendant?

A good local narc can easily average an extra $5,000 – $10,000 a month, or more, so why not get it while you can?

The problem of always coming in contact with valuable drugs, keeping some around for trading and authenticity, leads some narcs to reason, why not make a little profit at the same time? Local narcs (of course, this varies from place to place) aren't always subject to the same stringent check-in-and-out-or-explain-what-happened-to-it-rules about drugs as the Feds are.

Now and then, the major portion of a stash will not end up in court.

FEDERAL

Up until June, 1973, four separate government agencies were involved in the fight against drug abuse: Customs, Office of Drug Abuse Law Enforcement, Office of Narcotics Intelligence, and, of course, the good ol' Bureau of Narcotics and Dangerous Drugs.

These four agencies have now all been combined into one agency, under the attorney general's office, called the DRUG ENFORCEMENT ADMINISTRATION. The acting chief of the D.E.A. is one John Bartels.

This is good for those that applaud the drug control business, and bad for those who used to look forward to the various jealousies and guarded information and policies of the former agencies, which periodically resulted in humorous mess-ups and occasionally, at least in one instance, the shooting of a "suspicious character," who turned out to be another agent on the same case.

Narcotic assignment is a hazardous assignment, and rookies are garnered from all sizes and shapes of willing bodies. The major import is the ability to fit in with the drug community in physical attributes and ethnic persuasion. Local department narcs usually operate on a volunteer basis on the thought they perform better

WHAT'S WRONG WITH THIS PICTURE?

Can you find five things wrong with this picture? Can you find five things right? Can you pick out the narcs in the crowd? You can win. Or, you can lose.

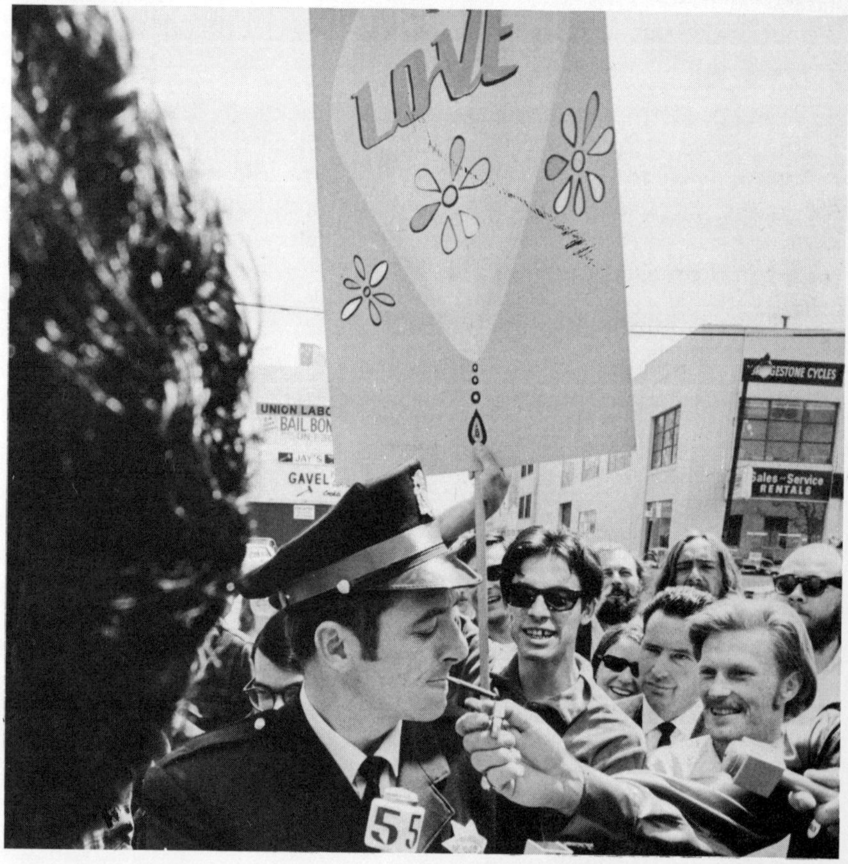

One of the heroes of the Hashbury days was Sergeant Sunshine, a San Francisco cop who became upset at a system where you could easily buy a gun but get arrested for smoking a harmless vegetable. On April 14, 1968, Sgt. Richard Bergess demonstrated his feelings by lighting up a joint on the courthouse steps. Hippies threw a carpet of flowers before the cop, who was promptly arrested by agents in the crowd. Needless to say, this was Sgt. Bergess' last day with the San Francisco police.

ELVIS PRESLEY RECEIVES HIS OWN NARCOTICS AGENT BADGE

Washington – Elvis Presley has been issued a narcotics badge by order of President Nixon. Presley was so overwhelmed by this action that tears sprang from his eyes and he hugged the president.

Presley was asked to cooperate with an antidrug campaign by the Federal Bureau of Narcotics and Dangerous Drugs. He agreed to cooperate and attempted to donate $5,000 to the bureau, which was refused by the bureau deputy director, Finlator.

Presley then asked if he could have a badge.

Finlator refused, saying he "absolutely could not let him have a badge."

Presley said he had an appointment with the president and he would ask him for a badge.

Finlator agreed saying, good-naturedly, "that's the only way you'll get one."

When he met the president, Elvis asked for the badge. "See that he gets it," replied Nixon.

Elvis reportedly was so overjoyed, he hugged the president and his eyes became misty.

than those who are ordered to do so. Federal narcs, on the other hand, are a different breed of cat.

An agent enters the esteemed service at one of two levels of civil service: GS-7 or GS-9. To enter at the GS-7 level, one must:

1. Have a bachelor's degree or three years of reasonable experience; or equivalent combination; AND

2. An appropriate qualifying score on the Federal Service Entrance Exam test; AND

3. One of the following: A. one year of graduate study.; B. one year of responsible experience.; C. any equivalent combination of A and B; or D. a 2.90 grade-point average on a 4.0 grade system OR rank in the upper third of your class OR membership in a national honorary scholarship society (other than freshmen or sophomore societies) recognized by the Association of College Honor societies.

To enter on a GS-9 level, one must establish eligibility on the mid-level examination (MAST) which has the same basic requirements as GS-7 level plus one of the following:

1. Completion of all requirements for an LL.B. degree or J.D. degree.

2. A master's degree or two additional years of full-time study in graduate level law enforcement, police administration, criminology, or directly related fields, OR

3. Two years of criminal investigative experience at a level equal to GS-7.

Narcs undergo a formal training period in Washington, D.C., which includes ten weeks of intensive training in such things as firearms, laws, courts, investigative procedures, drug ID, self-defense, etc. Each year they get a refresher course.

You must be 21 years of age to become a member of the DEA team, and you can hope for advancement to GS-9 at one year (or GS-11 if you started at 9). Then up to GS-12 based upon performance records. Management positions, when you are too old to operate effectively in the field, are at GS-13.

Agents are given two to five weeks vacation (paid) annually, depending upon length of service and are allowed 13 sick-days leave per year, plus nine paid holidays a year. You can look forward to a liberal retirement plan after 20 years of service.

On the bad side, you must be able to be reassigned anywhere at anytime, as workload determines the placement of DEA agents.

WOULD YOU SELL THIS MAN DOPE?

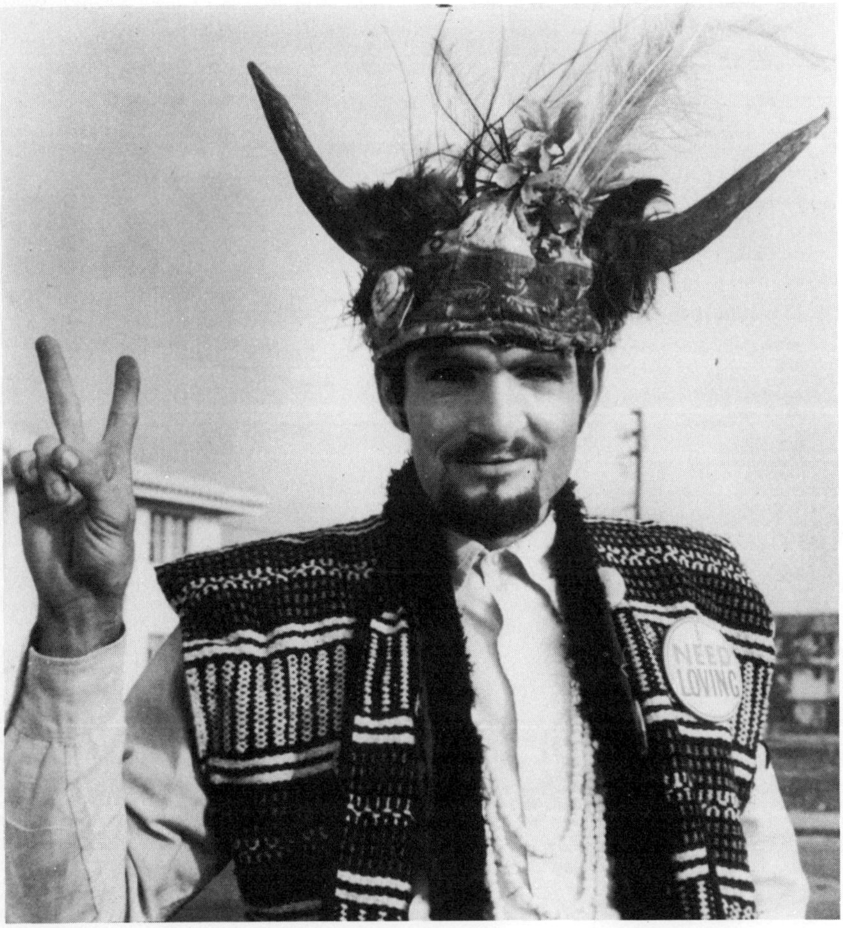

MIAMI, FLA., April 23 – HIPPIE AN UNDERCOVER COP – Giving a hippie sign meaning, "I have pot" is Miami Patrolman Bill Riley who has just completed a seven week assignment as an undercover agent mingling with hippie groups. A series of raids on psychedelic shops in Miami resulted from Riley's work. He is a Green Beret veteran of Vietnam and the beads, beard, jacket, and headdress were a part of his costume.

Photo courtesy of World Wide Photos.

Most narcs don't have to be too bloody clever to score – case in point:

Eduardo Bazua was arrested in San Francisco after he tried to sell an undercover agent 12 ounces of heroin for $17,000. The agent met Bazua at a corner gas station – Bazua didn't want to consummate the sale there. Wasn't there somewhere cool they could go?

What does the agent do? He hasn't planned on this, doesn't have any safe spot under surveillance, really doesn't want to take Bazua home to the wife and kids, so. . .

They march down to the Federal Building at 450 Golden Gate Avenue. Enter the building, take the elevator up to the 12th floor, enter the U.S. Drug Enforcement Agency's office, pass under the outstretched eagle and mottos, pass the other curious agents, and enter an unused room.

Bazua hauls out the dope. The agent weighs it and arrests him.

GENERAL

Narcotic officers, be they federal or local, are often operating in a void. They do not completely fit into the street drug-oriented world and must often employ some artificial means to cover this deficiency. The average (but not all) narc has relatively short hair and lives in a middle-to upper middle-class neighborhood.

He does not want to grow shoulder-length hair and live in a near-ghetto neighborhood and hang out with freaks in his off-duty hours. To combat these traits, the narc may often employ a wig, or he may try and make his straight traits work for him in the deal.

A short-haired narc may encourage the reputation that he works for/with the "Big Time" game; i.e., the Mafia or other unnamed, monied organizations. This evokes respect, fear, as well as explaining his age and physical features and gives him a solid reason for being interested in illicit drugs.

Narcs rarely ever operate alone, and Feds may function in groups of up to four or more people. Often only one may make the initial contact and then work the rest in as the partners with the money who want to meet the people they are dealing with.

Agents usually try and have the suspect on the hook before the final deal is accomplished. This is sometimes accomplished by asking for a sample which is RARELY ever consumed on the spot, but taken back to the "other partners" as the agent "doesn't like to talk business stoned."

The original "sample" can be used to force the dealer to stay in the game under threat of bust, if he gets cold feet.

Federal agents can usually only operate in one area until they are "made" by the dealing population. Then they are shipped to virgin territory.

Most initial contact is through "recruitment." That is, getting the goods on a small-time dealer, or if the agent is hard up, even a user, and letting him sweat in a holding cell for a while and then becoming a "friend" who will help him out of the mess if he will introduce him to the next step up the line.

This technique has been known to cause the most "hip" dealer to introduce the agent to his dealer or chemist as "a longtime pal," who the dealer has been selling to for years, just years, since childhood, you know. Now the new man wants to buy in larger quantities, and the dealer will turn him on to the chemist to save his buddy some money.

The variation on this deal is to make a couple of buys from a dealer and not bust him. The dealer gains confidence in his buyer (who often pays more than going prices) and will often introduce him to his contact as trustworthy on this basis. Dealers have the bad habit of exaggerating relationships of this sort. ("Man, I've done shit with this dude for years, he's cool.")

DEA people have access to a large variety of vehicles (many of which were confiscated in busts with dope or people containing dope in them – they are then passed on to the DEA to help with the image). Usually, these vehicles are registered to vacant lots, apartment houses, other nontraceable points to discourage dealers from discovering home addresses of narcs, although few dopers would have the sense to run down a narc's plate.

Federal agents usually arrange to have a few telephone numbers in the area they work, which are changed after major busts and ring in an office where either the agent or a nonsecretarial-sounding girl answers the phone with "hello." These numbers are given out to contacts as home phones where the dealer can reach the "buyer" when a good deal comes into town or when he finds his contact man and can arrange to introduce the "buyer."

When narcs stake out a suspect, they often use more than one vehicle and several agents, each of whom will take turns following the suspect in a different vehicle to make it harder to spot.

The average bust is made because of one glaring fact: most dope dealers are incredibly greedy and usually quite stupid in the bargain. They will happily take a buyer's word that "John Lake" is cool because John has flashed a bankroll and is from out of town and wants to buy a huge quantity at big prices because he can make so much more in Cleveland.

Most people get into the paranoia trip when dealing dope so heavily that they convince themselves the phone is constantly tapped by the FBI (a costly and rarer process than one might imagine), and people are always "watching" them. Usually they fail to notice anyone who is really watching them.

Dealers usually keep the dope in the same dwelling as they live to avoid "rip-offs," making it easy for a frustrated agent to simply get a warrant and march in finding the drugs scattered all over the place.

Agents sometimes have a limited amount of money budgeted to them for "buy" and cannot always come up with the entire amount should it run into the thousands. This is solved by padding a briefcase with money and putting the dealer in the position of feeling incredibly stupid and untrusting by asking to count it before the actual deal, or by showing a percentage of it and explaining the rest is produced when they have the dope in their possession.

Agents have access to almost any ID, but will not often leave their guns behind during a transaction. A mutual personal search before any dealing will often answer any questions about the authenticity of the buyer. (Although, this usually ends up in the agent walking out cussing the "shitty attitude" of the dealer, or the agent pulling his gun on the spot, especially if "samples" have been previously given or the agent knows the location of the dope.)

Of course, not all agents act this way. There are agents who are dirty, grimy, ride motorcycles, and live in the Haight, and might indulge in a bit of dope, if the time and situation calls for it. These are often the best agents.

Agents are only human, and it's no doubt happened that a narc will hold back some of a bust for later sale, but agents are watched by other agents, fairly closely, and are generally unbribable (federal agents, that is) and, generally, straight, although a narc will trade drugs, or give, maybe even sell drugs to the contact to win his confidence. (This dude must be cool, he sold me the first batch, you know.)

Dealers tend to play the role, use their real names, travel or dress flashily, travel in the same areas, carry the drugs on them, are greedy, don't really pay any attention to whether or not they are being followed.

Narcs are smart, do not use real names (except on court papers, by which time, it's a bit late), don't stay in the same area, travel with a backup man, are well-versed in prices and hip jargon and will bargain with the best buyer, are clever and good at their work.

Since the average seller follows the same personality traits, acts in the same stupid manner, sends drugs through the mail, talks about drugs all the time, etc., the narcs get a bit careless. When they come up against someone who doesn't use or dress like a dealer, uses several fake names, carries no drugs, checks alibis and license numbers of buyers, and doesn't trust anyone over 30, things can get a bit rough.

This is why there are so many more busts of the lower level dealers. Although the agents would greatly rather bust the chemists,

HEROIN HOTLINE

The toll free "hotline" established by President Nixon to encourage people to turn in (anonymously) pushers and other forms of lowlife has been a monumental failure.

In the first four months of the operation alone, the hotline program cost over a quarter of a million dollars and netted two grams of smack. Needless to say, at $125,000 a gram, this has to be considered a bit high priced, even for the media's idea of drug prices.

During this initial four month period, the line received over 28,000 calls, of which at least 24,000 were from phone nuts, hecklers, people wanting to get even with a friend or neighbor, or, as one official candidly put it, quite a few were downright obscene. . .

The most interesting call had to be from the San Francisco disc jockey who phoned in his (on-the-air) newscaster. He called back a few minutes later to report that it was a joke ("just to show the public how the line worked") and discovered that the hotline people lack any form of a sense of humor. . .the official became rather agitated, swore at the disc jockey, and informed him he would make sure his FCC license was revoked, and then he called the station manager.

smugglers, and quantity men, they have learned to avoid the stupid mistakes somewhat and are harder to pin down.

Most agents have nothing but contempt for the doper, his lifestyle, and the fact that he is selling drugs to other people. This hatred makes them more efficient in their job, often taking a bit greater risk than necessary, in order to get that big bust. However, it is always a game, they plan and probe, make contact and try to establish a buy—they can afford to be cautious. Sooner or later, the dealer loses.

SO YOU WANNA BE A NARC?

Here's a nice little training program for you.

The rookie is first exposed to experienced narcs to begin absorbing the actions and appearances of the role he is going to have to play. He is encouraged to join in "rap" sessions with the other officers to begin the transformation into a narc from a straight.

He is shown the "new" language that he must become familiar with and put at ease in the drug environment. He is brainwashed into reacting like a real addict or user, rather than reacting like a cop.

Many units have the rookies join in with the trainers in acting out dramas of a bust situation with the reactions of the cop. He is then critiqued by his fellows.

Then he is assigned to an undercover narc and sent on the streets to pick up the techniques needed to handle the informer, make the buy, talk street, and so on.

The narc works with a backup team of at least two other narcs, at all times. These backup men are supposed to be on hand in the background to assist the narc whenever possible and to gather evidence so the narc can act upon it. Normally the backup team will make the preliminary investigation, and at the finish of the job, they will arrest the target.

The narc is operating in an environment where he doesn't know anyone or have the host of other information usually available to the officer in a victim-crime situation. He must develop a source of reliable information to analyze in his investigation.

The favored method is to cultivate a good informer. The informer may be busted and trying to work off his own case (FEAR MOTIVATION) or may come forward on a revenge trip because he is mad at a pusher, or may be a dealer himself, who wants to cut down on the competition and learn more about the narc units in his area at the same time.

The good narc realizes this and plays the role necessary to instill the informer's cooperation. Normally the narc will register the informer with the division office and sometimes the local D.A. This holds an additional axe over the informer's head. If for any reason the cop thinks the informer is not dealing straight, he will classify him as "unsatisfactory," and the pigeon will never work with the bureau again. He will probably stand trial on his case, if any, or will be busted if has not already been.

The informer is "set straight" after initial contact is made. He must NEVER lose sight of who is boss. He must be informed that if he continues to deal or use, he will also be busted. Once committed, the officer must instill a desire to keep the informer on the straight and narrow.

Because the informer is known and taken into the drug circles, he can introduce the narc as a friend or potential buy. He must, therefore, be reliable. It is usually the job of the backup to interview and select informers.

The informer must NEVER be allowed to learn the cop's real identity. The narc must pick a street name and identify and ALWAYS stick to it, as he will run across the people in the scene time and time again, and could easily have his cover blown through one false step.

The first meeting of the narc and informer is a decisive step and must be psychologically "right." A cool meeting place away from the drug scene and away from all law enforcement personnel and places is usually selected. The narc will "straighten" out the potential informer by the "who's-gonna-be-the-boss" routine and then begin his sales pitch. A good cop should be able to see what is motivating the informer and play up this role.

A NARC MUST NEVER BAD MOUTH HIS INFORMER! Always convince him that he is a "deputy" or "special agent," or a representative of the "people" helping to clean out the "bad" dealers from the community. He is not a fink, rather a positive image of the things he values.

The cop should let little details "slip" if the informer is obviously trying to pump him for information about the narcs in his area, etc., to strengthen his own game. String him along, without giving out any useful details. NEVER DISCUSS OTHER UNDERCOVER AGENTS! This can be gotten around by the ploy of "supernarc."

Narcs often encourage rumors of a "supernarc" in the area

by using one common name when busting or hassling suspects. This soon leads to rumors of a hated agent who is everywhere. The other narcs can then capitalize on these rumors by suggesting the dealer is working for "supernarc" or telling how they were almost busted by "John Lake" themselves and describing him to win the dealer's confidence.

This "paranoia" invoked by the agents that the dealer may be a narc, or that they will call the deal off should "John Lake" be seen in the neighborhood is a fairly common ploy and usually has the effect of the dealer trying to prove he is righteous and not worrying about the authenticity of his "paranoid" friends.

A good narc must be able to pass back and forth between the two worlds he occupies with no stress. He should never let the informer know if he has a badge and gun with him or where he has them located.

If the contact man is to remain active for more than a few days, the meeting site should be frequently changed with no pattern involved, this protects the identity of both parties and convinces the informer that every possible precaution is being taken to protect him.

As you walk the streets, you should have the informer point out any neighborhood characteristics which could apply; i.e., dealer's houses, where alleys lead, where people hang out, what is the best way of the informer introducing the narc to the group, who is likely to get upset, etc.

When walking the street with an informer, the cop should keep him between himself and the buildings. This is a precaution and should trouble break out, the informer can be used as a shield. Should anyone attack the pair, he must first deal with the informer, which buys the cop a little time to make ready.

The length of time the officer has to remain on the streets varies with areas from a few minutes to several hours before the connection is secured and a buy made.

The informer should NOT be present during the transaction. A good way to handle this is for the narc to tell the informer to go watch for "pigs" while they make the buy. This usually makes the dealer happy, as he has one more lookout and one less witness. It is also necessary to make the informant a nonwitness so that he cannot be subpoenaed at the trial and his name does not have to be revealed, keeping him active.

A good pusher thinks he can always spot a narc and tends to

be overconfident, especially if the narc is introduced by a longtime buyer as cool.

The dealer may try several stunts to test out his new sale. He may ask to see tracks or suggest the buyer is a narc. The correct technique to apply here is to run a counterbluff. Accuse the pusher of being a narc or of trying to "burn" you. A different tactic is to agree with the dealer in a sugary sarcastic fashion. "Of course I'm the man. That's why I'm buying from a small-timer like you instead of someone worth busting."

The contact with the dealer should be kept to a minimum. The narc must get details to enable him to identify the pusher at a later date, but should give the pusher nothing to remind him of the narc later or remember him as anything but another buyer.

The first buy is usually fairly small as the narc is using public funds, usually which he has limited access to. The next buy can be a large one as the dealer now trusts the narc more, and the bust can come then, recovering any money brought along for the deal. The narc must never appear too casual about the money. It is sometimes necessary to flash large amounts ONLY TO SET UP A LARGE BUY, but he must never "front" the money, or act irresponsible with it, REAL DOPERS don't.

Most narc policies call for an initial buy and a break followed by a "B" buy at a later date. This serves several functions: it makes it hard for the pusher to come off as just a user selling to help a friend who asked him to, it gains the dealer's confidence, and it gets additional evidence and possibly new charges. The second bust can be much larger as the dealer now trusts the narc more, since he was not busted the first time.

If the second meeting is arranged before the narc has gotten a lab report back on the first buy, he must bluff his way through it. The dealer asks, "How was it?" A safe technique is to say, "not so good," or insinuate it was an outright burn. This puts the dealer on the defensive. He will try and convince you that you got his dope mixed up, or offer you more, perhaps of a stronger nature.

When a dealer admits he sells drugs to a stranger on someone else's word, he is vulnerable, and the narc can set him up at leisure.

If the buy is made in the room, the narc should always have the informer in a position to act as a shield when they first enter. He should immediately check out the room with regard to other people, possible escape routes, etc.

Often a wary dealer will suggest the narc use some of the dope

NO KNOCKING

Under normal circumstances, a narc must: (California State Penal Code)

1. Knock

2. Announce his presence.

3. Explain his purpose for being there.

4. Demand that entry be permitted.

The "no-knock" provision enacted by the U.S. Congress makes exception for these requirements ONLY for federal agents and under the circumstances where: a warrant has been issued, and it indicates that contraband is being kept in a place where it can and will be immediately destroyed if notice is given before entry.

It would take a RELIABLE source to indicate you keep your dope in a tissue wrapper perched on the back of your toilet.

HOWEVER, this can be ignored in circumstances where persons inside are KNOWN to be armed and dangerous.

As we go to press, it appears possible that the no-knock law will be modified, or possibly dropped altogether, as at least three cases of federal agents busting into the wrong homes have occurred within the span of a couple months. In every case, the agents, acting upon "reliable information," used the no-knock clause to break in without warning and spent the next few hours terrorizing occupants. In two cases, this meant normal, upright American families where the agents did such things as point a presumably loaded gun at the father and make him get on his knees while threatening to kill him in front of various members of his family.

In one case, the sole occupant was a pregnant woman who got the terror treatment.

The families received forced, belated apologies from the bureaus concerned, but they decided to file lawsuits anyway.

We will no doubt see at least a cooling off of the no-knock bit because of these suits and because the new DEA wants to establish a positive, non-Gestapo image.

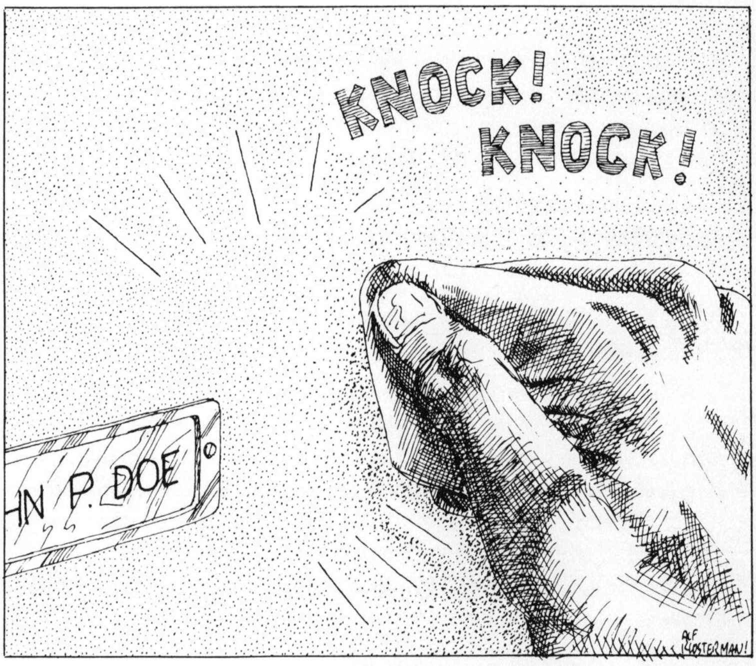

on the premises to prove himself or to see how good it is. A good cop forestalls this possibility by explaining the real money comes from his partner who wants the buy as a sample, or that he never deals when stoned, or that he and his "old lady" are going to use the dope later, together. If the narc fails to do this, he may find himself in the uncomfortable position of being "told" to do up some dope, possibly with several people around, waiting.

If the dope is hard, or even coke, the narc can possibly convince the pusher that he doesn't use anything stronger than grass or acid himself, or that the dope is for his friends or resale in a different part of the country, through his network.

If the offer includes shooting up, the cop can state he has had hep a couple of times and NEVER uses anyone's "works." If all fails, and he is told to shoot up or face trouble, he can:

1. Stall and wait for rescue by his backup unit.

2. Pull his weapon and make the bust then and there.

3. Fight his way out.

Of course, the stall is preferred. If the backup men bust a house, they ALWAYS arrest the narc along with everyone else. In this way he doesn't get identified as a narc.

After everyone is thrown in and booked, a detective will come along with a warrant for the narc on a much more serious charge somewhere else and make him go to serve out the other warrant. This way, the game is not blown, and the other dopers consider the narc a real criminal.

NEVER buy and bust a pusher. The narc should attempt to find out anything he can about the dealer; his street name, his real name, and where he lives, if he deals from the house, etc., while winning his confidence, so the bust can come later without blowing the narc's cover.

The narc gets introduced into a scene, establishes himself with the dealers, and begins making as many buys as possible from everyone that he can. After the "B" buy, the backup team comes in and starts arresting.

If the officer has accomplished his tasks of where the pusher lives, what and when he deals, etc., the busting is easy. The best busts take place at the dealer's apartment when the dealer is known to sell from his residence. If he deals mainly on the street, the "set" bust is the best as he is most likely to have dope on him at that point.

If a set bust is to take place, the narc normally signals his backup team who has the dope. This is often done by blowing his nose while talking to the target. The other narcs then move in and arrest everyone.

APARTMENT BUSTS ARE BEST DONE IN THE EARLY MORNING HOURS WHEN THE PUSHER IS STILL IN BED AND LESS LIKELY TO RESIST.

This is the most practical method of arrest in the terms of manpower and time, as the narcs choose the time and the place, and they don't have to wait for the pusher to make the first move. Usually they can find enough evidence (armed with the search warrant) to get other cases in the suspect's apartment. It is a good technique to get as many charges as possible for leverage with the judge.

It is common practice to throw the weight on to someone else after a quick bust. This is done by having an officer detain one of the pusher's last sales and allow the pusher to see him being "thanked" by an officer and sent on his way with no arrest. Another good idea is to drop a "careless word" about the source of information leading to the pusher's bust.

After the narc has made the bust, he returns to meet his covering team at a convenient location where they record the exact quantities of evidence which is then sealed and marked. He also writes down the details of the buy. The informant should not be present during this phase of the operation.

One of the problems of this sort of operation is that the officer cannot effectively penetrate the high school setting as his age difference is too apparent. The solution to this problem is to utilize young civilian police department employees as informers.

CONVERSATION WITH A NARC

The following is a verbatim conversation with a man who purported to be a federal narcotics officer.

Guide: Why did you become a narc?

Narc: I had just gotten out of school, where else could I have gotten that kind of bread with no experience? Besides, it's more exciting than working at a corporate job.

G: Do you consider yourself an average narc?

N: Well, that's a difficult question, you know, guys become officers for a number of reasons. I guess there's really about two different common varieties, those that really hate dopers with a fanaticism and those who are more in it for the excitement of the game.

G: Which are you?

N: I don't hate you.

G: Do you enjoy it?

N: Oh, yeah, sometimes you get a real smart pusher or chemist. It gets to be a real match of wits. That's the fun part. Most pushers are too god damned stupid to offer much of a challenge but occasionally you get a hot one.

G: Do you use any dope?

N: Ah, well, I've tried grass once or twice, but I don't use it. I don't really figure there's too much wrong with grass, but it would just be too hypocritical for me to use it and then bust people for it.

G: Do any narcs use dope?

N: Very, very few. Most stories you hear about officers keeping part of the stash out for personal use is pure bullshit. Sometimes, we'll keep a bit out for other purposes, to arrange deals and stuff.

G: But narcs have been known to steal money.

N: Shit, you bust up a pusher, who's been selling acid or worse to kids and he's got $5,000 cash, now are you going to tag all that bread and turn it in? You know where he got it. Officers are only human, you know. It's just part of the game, the fucking pusher knows he's running that risk.

G: Do you ever use your real name?

N: No way, never.

G: Are you married?

N: None of your business.

G: What do your friends think of your job?

N: The good ones don't care. Most of them consider it a public service. The acquaintances don't know. Besides, it's rough to build up any real friends that aren't with the department, because you move around a lot.

G: How often?

N: Oh, whenever you get known in an area. It could be as often as every six months.

G: Have you ever shot anyone?

N: No.

G: Have you ever had anyone pull a gun on you?

N: Yeah, in fact, once I got beaten up pretty good.

G: How did that happen?

N: Well, we were concentrating on this group of bikers that were making speed. I had gone in alone with about $2,000 to make a buy, and the backup unit had lost me, a fact which I didn't know at the time, and several more of the sonofabitches were waiting in the place. They jumped me and took the bread and worked me over pretty good.

G: Did they realize you were a narc?

N: No, they just figured I was some hippy-dippy dealer, and they would rip off an easy score. I didn't have any ID on me.

G: Did you catch them?

N: I didn't but several of my friends did.

G: What happened to them?

N: What do you think?

G: Do you make many grass busts?

N: Naw, we don't waste our time on grass except in large quantities, smuggling, growing, that sort of thing. It costs "x" number of dollars to make every bust, and it doesn't look good on your record if you use up all this bread and just get small fish, so we usually try and use small-time pushers and users to get one step up the line.

G: So you use informers?

N: Sure. That's where most of our busts come from. They're a funny bunch to work with. Most dealers figure they're safe if they just deal with friends, you know, but I have only run across a couple of pushers who wouldn't rat on their mothers to get a deal. They are usually overjoyed to introduce us as long lost friends to make a buy if it will save their skin a little.

G: So most informers operate from a fear motivation?

N: Fifty-fifty. You'd be surprised how many people are on this power trip, really want to bust other people just for the thrill of it. Also, some dealer will have a territory pretty well sewed up, and another dealer will move in, so he finks on the competition.

G: And you take a dealer's word for it?

N: Well, we check out every tip. Sure, we know it came from a doper, but the circle always turns, we'll get him in the end,too.

G: Wouldn't you say the average narc is on a power trip?

N: Oh, sure, some are. There's no doubt some of them get a bit carried away at times, but a lot of them really hate dopers and pushers, especially those with kids.

G: Have you ever lied on the stand?

N: Well, you've got to qualify that a bit. I've never lied to get anyone in trouble who was innocent, but I might have stretched the things a bit if the s.o.b. was guilty and might get off because someone forgot to label something just right or some other technicality some smart-ass lawyer brings in.

G: Doesn't this make you judge and jury?

N: Nooo, the jury doesn't know what went on. If I catch this guy red-handed and he's costing the taxpayers a fortune for a jury trial, and his lawyer is twisting the truth, well, shit, I might do it a bit also.

G: Don't you have to have collaborating testimony?

N: There are very few officers that are going to agree with a doper over a fellow officer.

G: Esprit de corps, huh?

N: (Laughing) Yeah, sort of.

G: Don't you ever have second thoughts about busting someone for smoking a vegetable?

N: No. It's the law that was passed by the people. If they make it legal, I'll be the first to stop harrassing them.

G: Would you use it?

N: (Laughing) I don't know. I've always been a Scotch man myself.

G: Do narcs ever take payola?

N: Definitely not. We are watched too closely to be fucking around. Oh, I am talking about federal now. You realize there are an awful lot of state and locals kicking around to qualify a statement like that. But, shit, I've personally handled over a million dollars worth of heroin that my backup and I could have turned over with no one being the wiser. Why would I take a couple of thousand to keep you out of jail?

G: Is there a lot of jealousy between the local units and the Feds?

N: There is a bit. No lie about that. We can't give up all our hard-worked-up information to every local cop who wants to make a big bust, too many leaks. If we are both working on a big case and it's about to break, there may be a bit of rivalry. Locals make more small-time busts, keep the pushers a bit nervous. We prefer to work behind the scenes a bit more and get the bigger fish.

G: What problems does the department face as a whole?

N: Believe it or not, we have always had trouble getting money to make buys and use for show (Ed's note: to flash to convince dealers that they really want to buy, not money to spend). "Buy money" is the taxpayers' and it's not usually recovered. We have to account for every bloody cent of that. Although Nixon has loosened this up somewhat. Lots of officers rely too heavily on disguise because they don't want to have to go home at night and face their neighbors with long hair and a beard but that never bothered me. I like looking funky (Ed's note: he did, too). Every bit of this hair is mine, all mine. Besides, it's harder to tell my age this way. That's something that works against every officer. You can only hit the streets for so long and then it's office-ville.

G: Are you experienced in any martial arts?

N: The department gives you a cram course, you know, plus, of course, we keep our marksmanship up, but I happen to be a black belt in karate. Some of the officers are just plain mean street fighters. Most all are pretty handy.

G: What do you do when you bust someone?

N: I pull my gun first, before identifying myself, before anything. Get that gun out there. Then I flash some ID or say I'm a police officer. You can watch the victim go through the changes. First, he sees the gun and figures it's a rip-off, and he looks around to see how he can jump me. I give 'em the ID bit and he always turns white. I guess prison flashes before his eyes or something, then he looks around for a way out.

I usually reinforce things at this stage by telling him he's a dead man if he so much as moves a muscle and then snap on the cuffs. All the time I keep threatening him with the mean act.

G: So, the idea is to keep him scared, right?

N: That's the whole philosophy in a nutshell, fear. . .

WHAT TO DO WHEN ARRESTED

If stopped on the street, be polite and RESPECTFUL. Cops search for weapons by patting down clothing, but you do not have to answer any questions other than your name and address. Innocent or guilty, DON'T SAY ANYTHING UNTIL YOU HAVE SEEN A LAWYER; EVER – NEVER –.

If you're in your home when the police arrive, do not consent to a search unless a search warrant is presented. If they ask, "can we come in," or "can we look around" and you wish to take the "I've-got-nothing-to-hide" attitude and say "surely" this is permission for a search, and anything found can be used against you.

If you are arrested, you will be told your rights and must be advised of the charge. It makes no difference if he really tells you this or not, if he says he did in court, he did.

If you are arrested illegally (a warrant with someone else's name, for instance) go along anyway.

If the cop is abusive and attempts to provoke something, BE CALM. Don't be a wise guy under any circumstances.

If you smart off and the cop beats you up, he will attempt to make it appear that you were injured in some other manner. An amazing number of abusive suspects fall down stairs on the way to being booked; or he will bring charges against you for resisting arrest and/or assaulting a police officer. No judge will believe he started it.

When you're arrested, note any details; the street you're on, look around for any witnesses, get the badge number of the arresting officer, write down any of this information that you can as soon as you have a chance.

The first rule of survival is GET A LAWYER! ! !

You will be booked and thrown in. Be sure you get a receipt for anything they take from you.

You are not required to give them any statements or sign any that you do give them.

On small crimes, the police will set bail; on larger crimes, the judge will. He has the right to set the bail almost anywhere he wants to, to insure you will show up for the trial. He will take into account how long you've been at your present job, your previous record, how stable you are, if you own property in the area, etc.

The bail bondsman will usually charge 10 per cent of the bond for his fee in putting up the entire bond. He can legally ask for anything for security, up to the full amount of the bail. He does not have to take the case. Bail bondsmen have an interconnecting network among themselves. If you skip, the police will visit the obvious places and then stop looking for you, assuming (usually correctly), you'll be picked up on something else and returned.

Bail bondsmen don't stop looking. They often find fugitives better than the police do.

PUSHERS – CORPORATE AND OTHERWISE

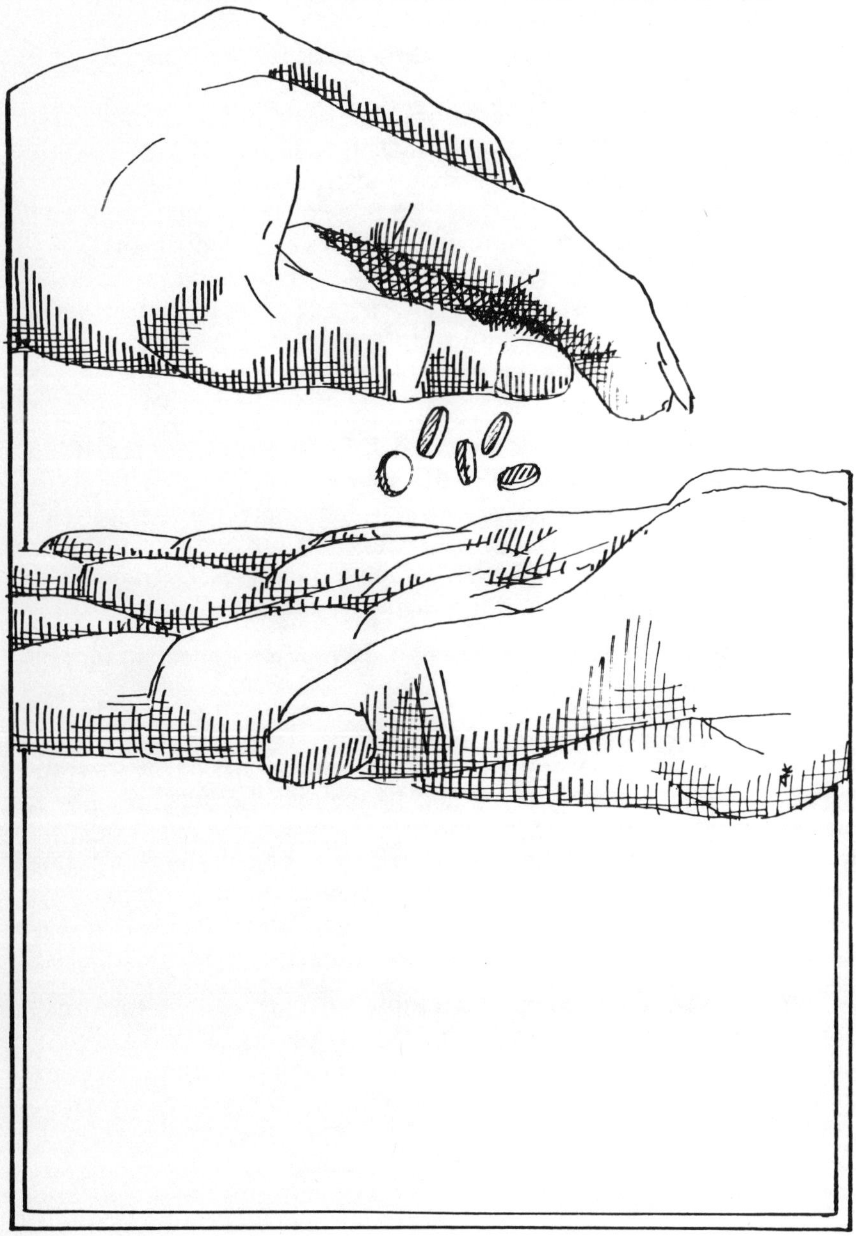

PUSHERS – CORPORATE AND OTHERWISE. . .

One of nature's least understood animals is the vivacious, red-breasted pusher. Some segments of society consider the pusher to be a nebulous ever-hatted creature who lurks around playgrounds ready to pounce on little kids and shove lighted reefers in their thrill-seeking mouths. . .On a general basis, society (i.e., in this particular case, the word "establishment" would draw a clearer picture, but I have dreaded that particular semantic gesture ever since it was discovered that FBI infiltration was the only thing keeping the SDS alive) tends to view the pusher as some sort of general, slime-covered lowlife who makes a hell of a lot of money by selling illicit drugs, tossed in with an occasional rape or burglary to stay in shape.

People who have had their apartment, or head, ripped off by one or more junkies, or have discovered their junior-high-school-aged kid is hooked, tend to feel that all pushers should be locked up for life with the proverbial key thrown away. In fact, New York seems to feel this way on a universal basis – that is, until they discover that it's their 10 year old who has been supplying the local sixth grade with reds ripped off from daddy's medicine cabinet. . .

Who are pushers? What do they do? What are the economics of the whole thing?

Figure that your "average" pusher started out as a user of one or more drugs and gradually worked into selling parts of his stash to friends. Sometime around this point, he realized that he could pay for his own drugs and make a bit on the side by buying in larger quantities and reselling to more and more "friends." The average small-time pusher is a college student (or high school or junior high school, etc., etc.), or other person who has ready access to a large number of people who are likely to share his enthusiasm for drugs.

Now, as the user begins to sell more than just enough to cover the cost of his own drugs and begins to get into the "support your lifestyle" syndrome, a few changes often come about. The pusher, or small-time dealer often discovers he has a sudden source of social desirability and power; people know his name, look for him and cultivate him for a friend. He gets invited to parties, meets new friends, and discovers that he now possesses a bit of charisma. Now, don't get

WHO CAN YOU TRUST?

Another problem with the dope scene is the fact that you just don't know who you can trust, know what I mean? For instance. . .

The mayor of Stow, Ohio, turned his 19-year-old son over to the local police for allegedly giving his other son marijuana. This crime falls under the giving-grass-to-a-minor act, punishable by up to 30 years under Ohio state law.

Mayor Howard learned of the alleged crime and couldn't sleep. Finally, at 3 a.m. he could stand it no longer and went down to turn his son in "for his own good."

The 19-year-old remained in Stow jail under $5,000 bond until his trial.

He was found innocent and released.

me wrong, the new-time pusher is not in a class with a real, honest-to-god rock musician, or something like that, you know, but he is definitely taking a step upward in the local pecking order.

This promotes a vicious circle of getting treated like something really hip and wanting to live up to the image. Pushers will often attempt to move up in the hierarchy of the whole thing by becoming "dealers" instead of "pushers." The new step implies that they are getting heavy, buying in larger quantities. ("Shit, a lid, man you must be kidding, I never sell no lids, man, I don't even sell single pounds!") He starts to live the role; neat clothes and/or cars, little gold spoons around the neck, fancy jewelry, shag haircuts, and all the time dropping names of how he's just one step away from the chemist. . .

As for money, well, everyone makes some, but the higher the level of operation, the greater the risks (along with the larger profit margins, of course). As the pusher gets larger, he may begin fronting dope to people who cannot afford to pay him in advance. He becomes a likely target for a rip-off (pushers and dealers are notorious targets for rip-off artists – are they going to run to the cops?), and, of course, the more people they deal with, and the larger quantities they sell, the more obvious they become to the narcs. . .

As a general rule, most pushers and small-time dealers make enough to live on, but many profits are wiped out by the rip-off here, the guy working for you gets busted with 3,000 hits of fronted acid there, the paid-for-in-advance dope comes out a grade or two lower than expected, etc., etc., etc.

However, pushers are universally working on that one big deal, the one that is going to make them $50,000, and then they can quit for good – the one that just never quite comes off. . .

As a small-time pusher does not get busted for some time (because of the sheer numbers of other small-timers and the fact that the Feds do not really want the little guy except as a setup to the big guy, and the locals just sorta take what they can get. . .), he becomes overconfident ("man, I know every narc in town, I can smell them. . ."). In reality, this situation allows the narc plenty of time to safely infiltrate the whole situation and get all the evidence that he needs for a secure case before busting anyone.

When pushers do become paranoid, they usually get excited at the wrong things. Almost every doper has felt sure that his phone is tapped at one time or another. He will believe rumors that so and so is a narc, rumors that are often started by rival dealers or even by narcs who wish to create a diversion and cover their own tracks.

In reality, the pusher should be suspicious of the people he deals with, i.e., his "friends"; this is especially true when any "friend" gets picked up and/or busted but not immediately sent up because of some likely sounding legal complication, or "probation". . .

Eventually, most pushers want to move up in the scheme of things to the point of being a large dealer, or even to the smuggling/ chemist level. This usually results in a pusher or small groups of same laying out money and time in a venture which they know absolutely nothing about. Seldom do people involved with the dope scene even take the time to investigate a grand-sounding idea as much as a normal, straight businessman would before investing money, and the doper is risking far more than just money.

Most dealers who decide to become smugglers or chemists usually accomplish nothing but doing some fairly stupid thing right off the bat, which throws the DEA spotlight right on them. It is fairly easy for the narcs to figure the moves from there on in. . .

Prospective chemists and dealers often write to various chemical companies for catalogs and then attempt to order necessary chemicals along with nondrug chemicals and equipment. THE CHEMICAL COMPANIES TURN THESE PEOPLE IN! ! !

Often, the bureau will authorize small sales and then photograph and trace the people who pick up the order. . .Phony explanations about why you are using the vacuum pump or the P_2P don't help. . .

Another bad one is buying gelatin capsules or large quantities of cutting materials such as Similac. In high drug areas, the druggists are told to inform the local agents when attempted (or successful) buys are made.

In one instance, the chemist of a local drug organization first discovered the agents were onto his phony chemical company by attending a lecture by the local police on the drug problem in that town. Someone asked about THC, the cop explained how it was very difficult and expensive to make, but then added that someone who they were watching had ordered the necessary chemicals just a couple of weeks before, and apparently was going to try and make it. The narc went on to explain the whole structure of the phony company and how they were going to bust them pretty soon.

Another drug group that had taken its name from a character in a famous novel was startled to read of its activities in LIFE Magazine before they had any idea that the authorities were on to them.

What it boils down to is: Most pushers and dealers dress flashily, use their real names, dig the heavy role and might as well be wearing little signs on their backs reading "arrest me."

Most narcs are trained, reasonably intelligent, and have nothing but time on their side. Guess who usually wins?

Now, there are exceptions, certain dealers, chemists, and the like have been operating for years, dealing only with a certain select group of clients, living with certain ground rules, and appearing straight for years, and have a hell of a bank balance (by the way, not kept in an accessible-by-the-authorities bank account). These guys are smart, and usually only take a fall for a couple of reasons: someone under them gets busted and snitches — this is the far-and-away number one reason for people getting busted. The guy can be cool for years, get one night in a 5 x 10 jail cell and rat on his mother, or they slip up, get tired, and break one of their ground rules "only just this once."

Many dealers know if they get hot (I mean, if someone is following you everywhere, it is probably a good time to think about retiring), but will continue anyway, "just for a little while, until the one last deal goes through". . .BINGO!

One friend of the author's did a solid acid and coke trade for years, always dealing in the same manner with the same people, never selling anything but the best, never ripping off anyone, driving an old car, dressing fairly cool, and working with only established organizations. At one point, some blacks observed him for a while, broke in and robbed him of several grand, a good, good stereo setup, some coke, and several pounds of grass, pistol-whipping him in the process. Another time, he was ready to leave for a trip to cool it for a while, when a long lost friend who needed just one little ounce of righteous coke showed up and was willing to pay a good price. . .

"Naw, I just don't want to sell anymore, I'm leaving town, I'm all done." (Now, this was a real friend, but not someone he usually sold to.)

"Please man, please as a personal favor, I really need it."

"Well, I'm leaving town in a day anyway, and well, I do still have a couple of ounces. . ."

"Far out man, I'll be back with the bread this afternoon."

That afternoon, the dude showed up with a "friend."

"Hey, this is uncool, I'm sorry, I never talk to strangers. I'm splitting for a while, see you in a couple of months. . ."

"Wait, wait, please man, this is a friend of mine from college, he was my roommate, I've known him for years, he has the bread and you can understand he doesn't know you and wouldn't front me the bread. He's cool, please man, I really need the coke. . ."

"Well, just this once, for you." Out comes the coke and out comes the badge. . .My friend's "friend" is just as astonished as he is. His "college roommate" turns out to be some guy whom he met a couple of months ago that offered him a free gram for turning him on to an ounce and would make him rich, and suggested not scaring his friend by saying he'd only known him for a couple of months.

Results: One year in county with the help of the most famous dope lawyer in S.F. ($3,500); a lost stash; a lost couple of grand, which the arresting officers confiscated, but never made it to court; some clothes; some camera equipment; and the end of a friendship. . .

Okay, now from the establishment's point of view. What do we do about this terrible menace, the pusher? Well, personally, I go along with the generally accepted Republican viewpoint — put 'em in jail for a few years, that'll learn 'em. Every time we pick up some kid selling coke, put him away for life, just like they do in New York.

Now, in all fairness, every time we pick up a batch of speed coming through customs, which some chemical company has mailed to a post office box in Mexico, where it doesn't take a federal license to order such things, and is being shipped back to the streets of America, just like the officers of the company know it is, we pick up the president of said company and put him in for life too, right? Next time, we go down to the first vice-president. . .and every time some freak gets arrested for pushing Quaalude, we bust the doctor who wrote the prescription for him for 300 tablets (like enough to put the city of Detroit to sleep for Lent) in there with him, right? Then we go back up the line to the company that made 50 per cent more Quaaludes than are being legally consumed AND KNEW ABOUT IT and put the remaining officers in jail for life, too, right?

Damn right, we'd clear up the drug problem. Besides which, we would stimulate the hell out of the economy, make major corporations places where junior officers could look forward to early, early promotions, give the cops something to do, and generally make prisons one hell of a lot more interesting places to be.

THE BROTHERHOOD

The "Brotherhood," a worldwide collection of dope dealers, which has reputedly been operating since the early Haight Ashbury days, has bitten the dust.

This nebulous organization dealt in a number of drugs, with the emphasis on grass and acid. They imported, manufactured, and sold their wares in all parts of the United States, and occasionally, overseas.

The "Brotherhood" also operated a number of successful, legal businesses to cover their interest in the drug scene, including several head shops and related "hip" trades on the West Coast.

The leaders of the Brotherhood supposedly included such drug "stars" as Stanley, the man, Owsley.

The Feds have pretty well busted and disbanded the Brotherhood through a long-term program of infiltration and information gathering, charging those caught in the act, so to speak, with drug counts and/or conspiracy and those not quite so sewn-up, with income tax evasion. Shades of Al Capone. . .

The IRS is still searching for at least six "leaders" who made good their escape to far friendlier lands, presumably with a large part of their ill-gotten gains.

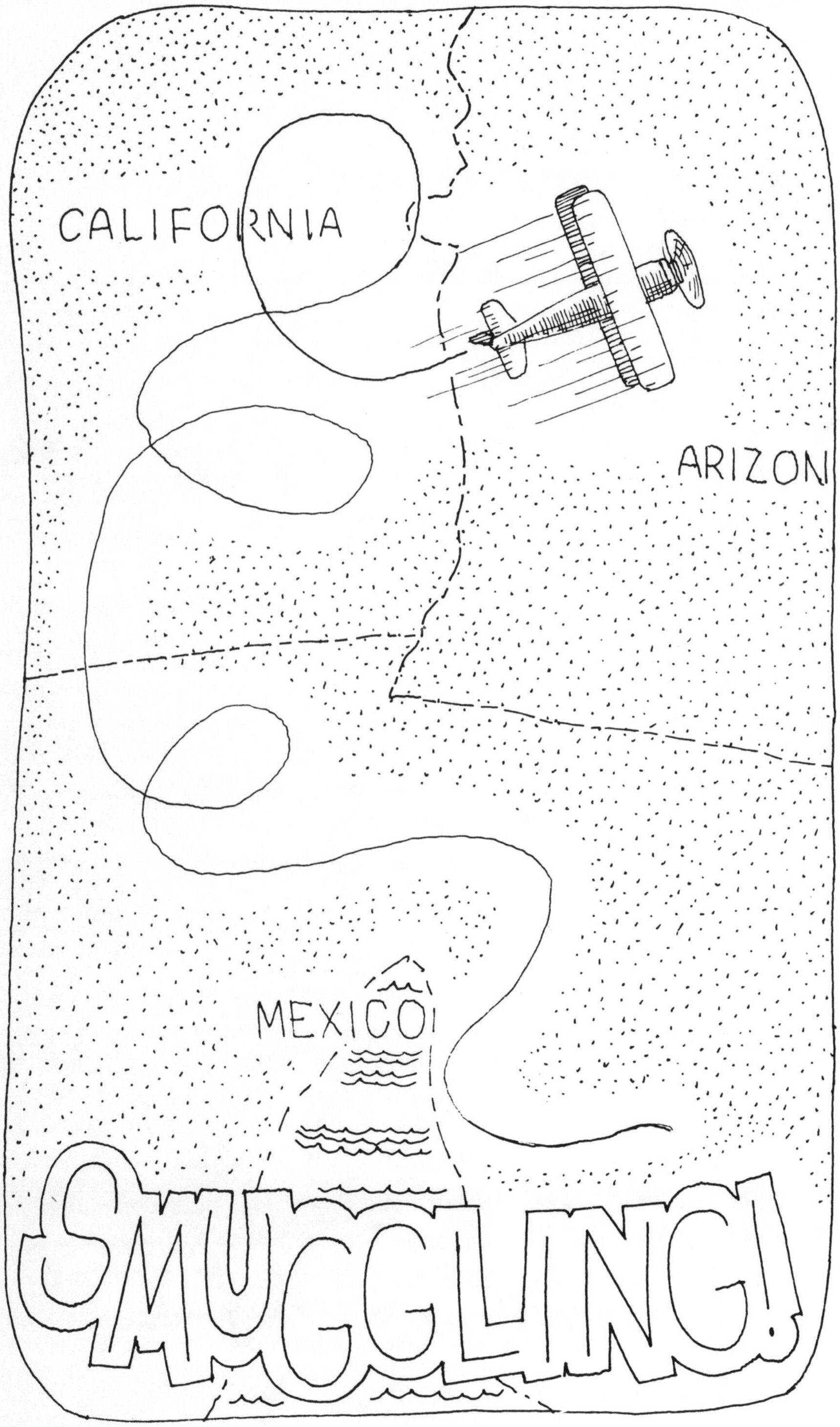
CALIFORNIA
ARIZON
MEXICO
SMUGGLING!

CONVERSATION WITH A SMUGGLER

Ed. Note: *"Bob Evans" is a New Mexico-based smuggler. He and his friends bring in some righteous grass from deep in the heart of Mexico. "Bob" is not, of course, his real name, as at the time we go to press, he is still active and happy. . .*

Us: Who smuggles?

Bob: Most of the people I deal with are dopers who are tired of paying rip-off prices for good dope. A lot of us are Army or Air Force trained.

U: What do you fly?

B: A Piper Aztec twin — fast cruise (around 250 mph) and good range. I ripped out everything that wasn't nailed down and installed extra tanks for long journeys. I've got several radios set on the various federal frequencies, but nothing else, unless it's essential.

U: How much dope do you bring back?

B: We average about 750 pounds on a good flight. We load it in duffel bags and stick cargo chutes on 'em.

U: Do you throw the dope out or land with it?

B: Both, try and vary the routine. We don't stay with the same MO more than twice in a row. . .

U: What's it like?

B: Oh, you know, we take off from a small field in New Mexico or Texas and stay low, hit the border under 500 feet to avoid the radar. A good trip involves going pretty far down, so we usually have one fuel stop somewhere along the way. We're lucky for a small operation; we've got good contacts.

We tripped down by van once and met some good front people, they're American. We pay a bit more for the dope, but it eliminates the biggest hassle of the trip, dealing with the Mexican suppliers.

You can't trust those guys. A few times everything goes hunky-dory, then they come out of the bushes shooting and bam! That's all she wrote. They're supposed to bring gas, but they're pretty unreliable. Sometimes, it's watered down pretty badly, or they forget.

I had one pilot who made the connection okay, gassed up, and found his engines wouldn't do it. Sons of bitches had loaded 'em with 100 per cent kerosene. . .He had to walk out and catch a ride back up. When we flew back down, no plane, no dope, nothin'. . .

There's quite a few wrecked or scavenged aircraft scattered around the desert down there. . .

U: What are the other hang-ups, border patrol?

B: Naw, those guys aren't too bad — understaffed. They're usually flying low looking over the border for wetback tracks. We get a few diehards, sure, but the worst are the Mexican Federales. Those guys have a real special place in their hearts for Thompson submachine guns. . .Like to fly right out of the sun on your blind side, kick open the door and start shooting. . .It's a real game to them.

We never go up without the guns. . .Can't chance mounted wing guns because we have to use commercial airports, but, we're never without a gun for every man aboard.

U: What do you pay for dope?

B: Oh, we average about $20 - $30 a key. Depends on quality, season, etc. We could go in cheaper, but more risky.

U: How big is your operation?

B: We run about two planes, sometimes more. We can always dig up an out-of-work pilot if we need to. Getting the plane is the problem. Some dudes rip 'em off and change the wing number. But all the border patrol planes have infrared detectors to spot altered numbers.

There are other people who are flying big loads, commercial operations every night with multiengined planes that can bring a lot of dope in on one shot. But that takes a lot of organization and a lot of payoffs and people keeping their mouths shut. We'll never get that greedy.

U: How many planes come over on a heavy night?

B: Maybe as many as sixty or seventy on a hot night. . .

U: Do you pay anybody off?

B: No, we don't. Some cats do. One operation I worked with for a while has a whole town set up for them. They've put money into the town, building a little hospital. The mayor helps them load it. The town loves 'em, the farmers sell to them only, everyone treats them like visiting royalty. . .

U: What do you use for landing strips?

B: Down there, we usually block off a road and use it. Not too much traffic where we are. When we come up, we hit one of the little, almost abandoned, fields in Texas. Emergency landing fields for the FAA. We come in low, do a touch and go, or even stop and unload, then head up into the radar and file a radio flight plan as taking off from that field. We usually head right to a small airport and gas up and then head into Denver, Taos, or even Cal.

U: What kind of plane is ideal?

B: Well, it depends on what you want. We are primarily interested in long range and being able to outmaneuver the Cessnas the Federales use. A Constellation could probably bring in a quarter of a million or so each trip. . .I knew one crazy man who used his Lear jet. . .He'd file a flight plan on business, pick up the dope, and kick it out with cargo chutes just over the border.

U: Where are the big smugglers?

B: Oh, you know, Sausalito is a hot spot. There are bars there that almost cater to the Air Force. Pilots sit around and trade stories about the best strips, close shaves, etc. I read somewhere that Sausalito has more planes than most of the nations that sit at the U.N.. . .

Some of the big operations are using well over 100 planes. . .including stripped-down Constellations. . .

U: Why do you do it?

B: Well, there's no denying the thrill of setting up the operation. It can get pretty tricky, and it's better bread than we could make anywhere else. I really wouldn't want to sit in a Mexican jail too long, although we could probably buy our way out of anything deep inside. The border patrol would be a bitch, though. . .

U: Do most of the big operations bring in hard stuff or just grass?

B: Almost everyone brings back a little coke, mostly personal. Other than that, it's pretty much limited to grass. No pills, no smack, or anything.

U: What else do people use for smuggling?

B: There are some guys around, one group in particular, who is getting into some pretty wild trips. . .Radio controlled drone planes that can bring in one hundred pounds or so. They fly really low, like under bridges and stuff. Most are short range, just for skipping the border.

One guy I knew was even trying hot air balloons. One shipment went fine, one the wind changed. I can still see that guy trying to shoot his balloon down, driving this CJ-5 over the desert with the balloon just outdistancing him. . .Never got it, either.

U: Is there anything else you do to the plane?

B: We try to make it as invisible as possible, both from the ground and from the air. Camouflage would attract a bit too much notice, so we do the upper half in brown and the bottom in white. Makes the plane pretty nearly invisible from either direction with the right landscape.

I usually take one other guy along. A copilot who could fly if I got shot up and who can handle a gun. I like shotguns, the Mexicans seem to respect them the most. It at least keeps them back a bit where their Thompsons aren't too accurate.

THE ART OF DO IT YOURSELF

The major word in do-it-yourself smuggling is — don't. Custom agents are not stupid or lax by any means, and while they are greatly outnumbered, (i.e. 600 customs agents for the state of New York versus 6,000,000 passengers a year through the New York entry points), they are also very professional.

True, thousands and thousands of kilos of illicit drugs are brought through or over the borders each year, but the majority are handled by professionals with a good organization behind them, and even they get busted.

A semilong-haired kid is going to get searched through customs. Period. That's all there is to it. If you are heavy, you will be busted. Customs agents miss very little when they have decided to search someone.

They are also hip to almost all the places for bringing in dope. It may seem very clever to sit around and think of putting some hash in your pack frame or putting some lysergic acid in the cologne bottle, but dig it, you stand a very good chance of going up — agents have seen ALL the hiding places and know where to look.

Also very overworked is the false bottom routine; the putting it in animal cages; making hash into statues or other "works of art"; filling hollow heels, sandal soles; sewing it into patches or cuffs; or stashing in the spare tire, ceiling panels, doors, air cleaners, or for that matter, anywhere in a vehicle.

A federal smuggling bust is not good. You stand a very good

chance of a 100-grand bond for a pound of coke and maybe fifteen long, hard years in the joint. Think about it.

Agents do use dogs at some points and at a couple, there have been reports of using electronic "sniffers," which can detect and analyze a few ATOMS of dope in the air. Very few things can be sealed tight enough to prevent this sort of leakage.

The best way to bring in dope, if you've really got the urge, is probably to avoid customs all together and just hassle with the border patrols, but success in this field requires as much or more organization, planning, and information (not to mention money) as trying to bluff it through customs.

The diplomatic passport route still works, to some degree. Agents will get permission and bust a diplomatic passport holder if they have reason to believe it is being used for illicit purposes.

MAIL

The mails still bring in a large amount of dope, but the Viet Nam "conflict" did much to cut this down. Many international receiving post offices use dogs, x-ray machines, and physical inspections. While not every package gets the treatment, packages to/from hot areas and people stand a much better chance.

Besides any super standouts, an inspector picks one out of every so many packages and opens it for inspection on a purely random basis. The law of shitty averages being what it is, your dope packages seem to get it more often than true percentage warrants on this kind of deal.

When dealing with the mails, you have an additional problem to worry about. Many P.O.s are staffed by young freaks who have the rotten habit of learning the usual places for dope and stealing any they can find before the inspector can get it. While this is certainly preferable to having a cop find it, it is still a loss.

Be advised, if they find dope in the mails, it will often still be delivered, after the narcs are notified, or course. They will follow the receiver and mark him or perhaps give him long enough to open it and dust him.

If you get a package of dope and open it and do not destroy it or call the police, you ARE guilty of at least possession and maybe worse.

The following letter is written by a former post office "freak":

As a former postal employee, I can attest to the fact that thousands of pounds of narcotics are safely shipped throughout the world via the U.S. Post Office. With the huge volume of mail handled each year, adequate inspections are impossible.

In preparing a shipment of dope to be sent through the mail, remember that the customs inspector is just doing his gig and wants to do as little work as possible. All mail coming into this country from abroad goes along a conveyor belt passed by an inspector. He is told to open every twelfth package or anything that looks suspicious.

In most cases, the inspector merely opens the package and looks inside. A hollowed-out statue filled with hash looks just like a statue not filled with hash. (So long as it does not rattle). A large chocolate bar interspaced with pieces of hash would not get a second look, as long as the wrappers did not appear to have been tampered with. An expensive book in a leather case would draw no attention, even though it might have a drop of acid on each page.

Anyone who thinks that writing three words on the outside of a package will cause anyone to handle it with any special treatment is still living in the dark ages. In shipping, you must take care to wrap each package well. Most illicit shipments are not discovered by the inspectors, but rather when they break apart due to the handling they receive.

Some customs facilities are equipped with x-ray machines, most are of poor quality and cannot see well through tin foil on the inside of the package.

They will not x-ray anything that says on the outside, "Do not x-ray — magnetic tape," or anything that says, "Film." They may open such packages to check and you had better have some film in there, or they'll tear the package apart.

If you follow these instructions, it's hard to get busted, but nothing is impossible. Many misconceptions about mail busts: One; they do not hold busted packages in the P.O. They rewrap it and sent it along its way, notifying the narcs in the addressee's area. Two; they cannot bust you when you go to pick up the package. They must be able to prove you knew there was dope inside. So, they wait till you take it home and have a chance to open it. If you leave it around for a few days unopened, and the narcs descend, there is nothing they can do about it. The only one that can open that package once it's been delivered is you. If you notice strange cars outside your house after you get the package, or if you feel the package has been opened, or you don't recognize the handwriting (sometimes, postal employees will readdress the package after resealing), or if you have any reason to believe that the package has been rewrapped, hide it. Dig a hole and bury it, throw it away, or let it sit on the shelf UNOPENED, until you are sure it's cool (usually about a week).

Some of the more imaginative shipments are found by mere coincidence. One of the classics was a box marked "urine samples," which actually contained vials of acid. For an authentic touch, the senders had spilled some real urine on the package to look as if a vial had broken open. No one even wanted to touch it, let alone inspect it. After a year of shipping acid this way, the P.O. got wise and hired an inspector to check all the urine samples, broken or not.

And now a word for our fighting men all over the world. Cassettes are the most effective way of doing your thing back to the States. All military mail facilities are equipped with x-ray machines, but x-raying cassettes would ruin them, so they are left alone. The best thing about cassettes is the sheer number of them. Thousands are sent into the States each day, and they are treated just like regular mail because they're so easy to toss into the right bin.

The important thing to remember when doing it with cassettes is the weight must match exactly with a real cassette. Be sure and seal it well, so it doesn't fly open, but don't use so much tape to be conspicuous.

A last word of advice to heed, or not, as you see fit, is to use your commanding officer's return address, and don't send it to your own home in your own name.

Although all the methods I've mentioned are good, the best thing to do is invent your own. Have fun, turn on your pen pals, but USE ZIP CODES.

GENERAL

There are several things one should be aware of when using, or smuggling dope in other lands. The first is that Americans have, very possibly, the shittiest deal going anywhere. On July 17, 1971 (I might add here, with a touch of irony, that is my birthday. . .) our beloved ex-President declared a total global war on drugs and drug people.

Since this time, America has poured millions and millions into bribing countries not to grow dope (although Turkey has just renounced the bribe and decided to grow opium poppies again), as well as providing "information, advisors, training, commodity and equipment support, and funding" to foriegn governments who wish to "develop effective drug law enforcement capabilities."

This translates as our government encouraging drug busts and to the point of scattering CIA agents around the globe to act as informants and "advisors" (remember Viet Nam?). These agents do not arrest directly, but do help local police accomplish the same end.

As one might hazard a guess, with America denouncing druggies the world over, she does not do much to help her own citizens when they fall prey to a drug bust. In fact, America probably does less than any other country to help arrested citizens. It has been rumored that America even ENCOURAGES harsh treatment in foreign (notably, Mexican) prisons, of American prisoners.

At least one person has died because an American embassy refused to help authorize treatment in a proper hospital AFTER THE HOST COUNTRY RECOMMENDED IT.

Add all this to the fact that many less "privileged" countries do not take well to "rich," long-haired, faggy-looking Americans, anyway, and you have the nucleus of a real problem.

Most people get busted for one of several reasons: they are under financed and/or too greedy, they trust the nice, long-haired freak who offered to help them out, they try to beat customs (rather than trying to get through lightly patrolled border regions), or they're just plain unlucky. . .

If you do get popped in a foreign land, the very least it will do is help you appreciate America a bit more. Many, many countries have severe sentences, miserable jails, physical confession inducements, and the belief that you are guilty unless proven innocent.

A few things to bear in mind are: NEVER, never, under threat of hanging from your thumbs for twenty years, sign any confessions or papers that you do not understand after being arrested. You will have plenty of time to think about what you want to say afterwards, believe me.

Never admit you have ever smoked dope: IN SOME COUNTRIES (as Turkey and Greece), THIS STATEMENT WILL SEND YOU TO JAIL FOR AT LEAST SIX MONTHS. NEVER SAY YOU SHARED OR GAVE DOPE TO ANYONE. Courts will give you much harder sentences if you passed a joint to a native and helped corrupt him, than if you kept it among your weird foreigners.

Always be humble and polite as possible when arrested. Do not answer any questions about your crime, BUT DO IT IN A POLITE WAY.

In some areas, a laywer can help greatly, some places, it is a waste of time and money. Talk to other prisoners, contact any groups (listed at the end of this section) in the area.

It must be noted that in many countries, MONEY IS A NECESSITY WHEN you are a criminal. Some places may let you off with a bribe, some will give you preferable treatment of reduced charges, and some will send you up anyway, but not beat the hell out of you daily if you pay the prison officials.

Mexico is noted for their shitty prisons and bribe system. A person in a Mexican jail can get food, get out of work, pay protection, and sometimes even get out early or arrange an "escape" with enough money. However, there are many rip-off "lawyers" and "friends" in Mexico who make a habit of contacting American prisoner's relatives in the States and offering release for a couple of thousand dollars. Usually, the money disappears with the "friend."

If you are driving a car and you are a "suspect," you can be stopped and the entire car disassembled. If any, and I mean any, dope is discovered, the whole vehicle is then cut up with torches, if necessary, to find the "rest." If you are convicted, your chances of getting the vehicle (and anything in it) back is about nil.

In many areas, where dope is easily available (Afghanistan, Moracco, Turkey and the like) the customs and local narcs will know what roads you are taking, and how long you spent in certain areas. If any time exceeds what they feel it should exceed, you will be stopped and searched unexpectedly.

A final word: many cops will use the "if you fink on one other person in your party, you'll go free" routine. BULLSHIT! Many will take both you and the person you pointed at and charge conspiracy and send both of you up for a longer stretch.

QUICK HARD SUMMARY

First of all, let me say that if you are going to trip abroad (pun intended) get a copy of the TRUCKERS BIBLE (see suggested reading list at end of book).

AFGHANISTAN

Money is very important. Potentials are timed at road checks and stopped and searched if the timing appears "suspicious." Many informers, you will be found guilty if arrested. Fine and sentence (figure under a $1,000 fine for fooling around, several for smuggling). If you pay up light sentence or release, without BLAM: Heavy time and rough prisons where you must BUY YOUR FOOD – or starve.

ALGERIA

Rough laws and rough police. Beatings and such are common. Some bribery and heavy time.

BELGIUM

Average sentences (six months to three years) but may get worse.

CANADA

Easier than the States. Generally a fine for first offense, less than one year for small sales and 7+ years for importation. Organized intelligent agents, no bribery, no physical abuse.

EGYPT

Oh yeah, figure up to 20 YEARS for "pushing," maybe life (although execution is on the books) for smuggling. Any drugs passing through (such as a flight change at an airport) is counted as THERE.

ENGLAND

Difficult to get bail (if you're not from England), may wait a long time for your case to be heard. Minor fines and/or a taste of time for possession; several years for smuggling. Legal aid available.

FRANCE

Heavy busts, seem to hit quite a few Americans. Small personal bits may get a "customs fine" and off or light sentence. Sales or smuggling will net a few years. Long waits for trials, some brutality from the friendly agents, heavy customs fines which are added to your sentence if not paid.

Most all baggage, including personal, is x-rayed. Be especially wary at the Spanish border.

GREECE

Ah yes, wonderful Greece, where thousands of young types go to enjoy the fun 'n sun. Wonderful Greece where if the local authorities feel you're helping corrupt the young (long hair, that sort of thing), you can/will be busted for smoking reefers, set up by one of the many local informers, or arrested (and convicted) on a purely bogus charge. Very heavy sentences, with all "narcotics" (including LSD, hash, grass, STP, codeine, demoral, etc., etc.) bring a MINIMUM of two years for possession and 5 - 20 years for sales, smuggling, receiving letters containing drugs, transport, and other biggies. Police brutality and anti-American sentiments.

HOLLAND

Fairly easy going. Light sentences of under one year for most small offenses and a couple of years for smuggling. Dogs at airports. . .

INDIA

Not bad, often reasonable fines rather than time. Possible deportation instead of jail, not too many arrests.

ITALY

Funny, hard to tell, May await trial for two years and then be deported. Good lawyer and bribe money can often help. Some of the Mexican "lawyers and friends" brand of rip-off artists around. Possession busts do occur for one joint.

JORDAN

Not too strict. Most busts are from luggage and other cheap smuggling attempts. Less than one year for under five keys of grass. A couple or three years for heavy smuggling. Foreigners can get reasonable bail.

KENYA

If dope busts are in vogue, expect a heavy fine and light time, otherwise, a light fine. Avoid lawyers. Dope is not considered too heavy of a crime, and you can often play it down.

LEBANON

Very good customs, quite a few Americans get popped here. Small, quantities (if you can convince them that it is personal) may get six months, IF THE CUSTOMS FINE IS PAID. Larger quantities get in the area of three years.

Many informers, much professional police brutality, and quick violence if you refuse to sign things.

LIBYA

BUMMER.

MEXICO

Many informers, rotten prisons, funny cops, and anti-gringo feelings. Bribery, once the accepted judicial system, is falling off in high places. Try to bribe the cop ASAP (if you're going to try it at all) before your case reaches a higher level. Money is a real necessity to avoid daily beatings in prison and get little luxuries like food.

MOROCCO

Heavy police activity, spot vehicle checks, rough customs, many informers, rip-off lawyers. Sentences are not among the worst, i.e., about one year for possession and two for smuggling. Bribery helps reduce sentences and money keeps your ass in one piece once you are inside.

NEPAL

At the time of this writing, they do have dope laws in Nepal, but they may lose them once again. At any rate, busts result in horrendous penalties, say $100 fines for smuggling. . .it is possible to spend a few days in jail if you blow it. Very bribable, dope is considered sort of an unofficial customs pension plan. . .

PAKISTAN

Pakistan WILL note your check points at customs and how far down the road you are in a matter of time. If the actual doesn't jive with the projected, stop and search. . .many informers. Much very organized smuggling goes on unmolested, so the little guy gets popped to keep up the facade. Not too bad sentences (One year sort of thing) weird jails with a caste system. . .money. . .money. . .money.

RUSSIA

Unless you are a Solzhenetsyn groupie and want to try out the local labor camps for two years to see if they're all they're cracked up to be. . .avoid dope in Russia.

SOUTH AFRICA

Eeek! Possible to get ten years for dealing, and god knows what would happen if you are black. Why go to South Africa anyway?

SPAIN

Ah yes, the DRIFTER's. . .glorious Spain. Beware of the airports, may check stop-over flights just for the fun of it. Customs duty is HIGH and WILL BE PAID or you will get another several years on top of your your six month upward use or three - six year smuggling charge. Some chance of deportation instead of time if it is a small bust, (under nine - ten keys), if you are not part of a "conspiracy", have money. . . good lawyer hard to find and very necessary. May wait six months for trial.

TURKEY

Bad news. Police brutality, heavy fines, three - five years for USE or small possession, up to LIFE for smuggling. Heavy blackmailing as police will cut people loose or return passports if you snitch on someone they want. A roach means two years in prison, simple as that. Police are often bribable, judges do not appear to be. . .

If you are busted overseas, get in touch with your consulate, which will do you absolutely no good except to tell the folks back home that you made it, and contact one of the groups here who may be able to at least help you select a good lawyer and give their condolences.

STREET DRUGS

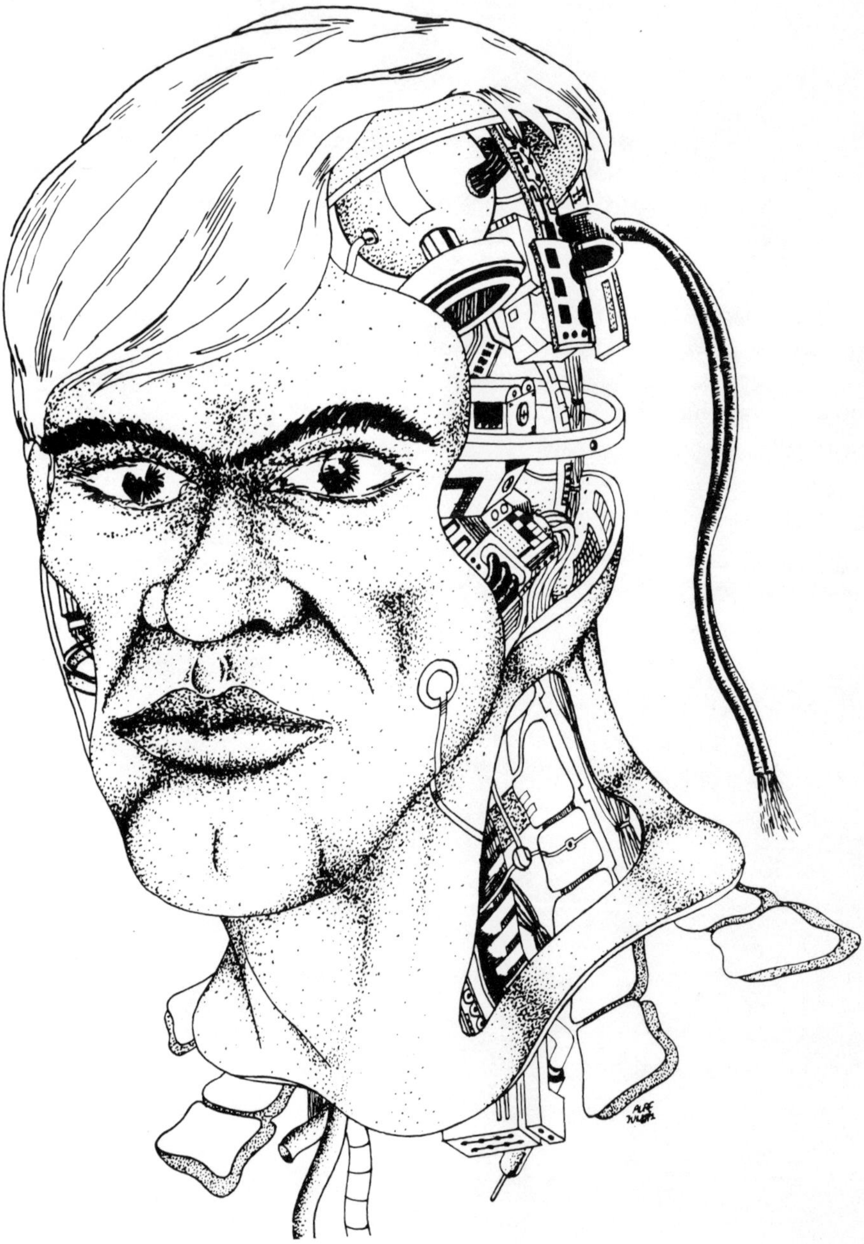

BARBITURATES

Nembutal — Yellow jackets

Seconal — Reds

Amytal — Blues

Luminal — Purples

Barbiturates are the most widely used depressant drugs available and the most misused. Medically, they are used for epilepsy, insomnia, and emotional disorders. A person on barbs will generally be sluggish, have slurred speech, and be very emotional, ranging from tears to laughter. He can get irritable and antagonistic, especially on any combination of barbs and alcohol.

ODing can occur because various types of barbs take longer to take effect and last longer, some will run 3 - 4 hours, some 6 - 8, and some over 12 hours.

The action of barbiturates and alcohol is addictive and depends on many variables: dose of both drugs, time for metabolism, etc. A safe dose at one time can be fatal at another, by overly depressing both the respiratory and cardiovascular systems.

More people die in the U.S. from barb OD than from all the other drugs combined, including smack.

BUFOTENINE

Bufotenine or 5-hydroxydimethyltryptamine is a drug which was first synthesized from the glandular secretions of toads. It is also present in cohoba and in the psychotropic mushroom, fly agaric. It is minutely present in banana skins.

Related to DMT, bufotenine is rarely found in America.

COCAINE

The early Inca Indians chewed the leaves of a strange plant to alleviate hunger, provide them with seemingly unlimited endurance, and make life a bit more bearable. Early tombs, which have been opened by prying archaeologists, have been found filled with coca leaves, presumably to give the dead something to do in the great pyramid in the sky.

American slave owners used to import the leaves to make the slaves work harder and eat less. Due to this practice, some states passed anticoca laws.

Then in 1866, the fun element in the coca plant was isolated. They named it cocaine.

Early coke was used as an anesthetic (local in operations) and gradually became the rage at parties around the "jet" set of the late 1800s.

Among other people of some note, Sigmund Freud became hooked on the habit and reportedly had at least three nose operations to combat the residual effects of the drug.

Coke became available in a variety of forms from medicine to candy. One famous cola drink was flavored with the good ol' coke plant. This was a stroke of genius, after all, what could be more in the spirit of free enterprise than a habit-forming soft drink? In those merry days, Coca Cola was the "real thing."

In the early 1900s, the government began passing around rumors of killing sprees and other criminal behavior caused by the evil drug, and in 1906 it was outlawed in the U.S.

GENERAL INFO

Coke is still used a little bit for medicinal purposes, such as plastic surgery, but it is impossible to obtain in a pure form under prescription. If it were possible, an ounce would sell over the counter for about $50. Hell, you might even get it for $35 in a discount drug center.

Coke alleviates fatigue and promotes work. It produces a characteristic speedlike high, without the wiring effect felt in speed. It heightens the sensations and at the same time numbs them to unpleasant sensations such as pain. It is widely used by those in the entertainment field as a crutch before shows or during heavy practice or recording sessions.

Coke usually causes some local numbing of the nose, mouth area, and teeth. The nose will start to run somewhere into the high and will quit as the high tapers off.

Heavy users tend to switch off with other drugs (downers to counter the residual excitability that is left over).

It has rapidly become the elite of the underground drugs. I mean, any fool can see what damage smack and speed do to a person, but coke, ah, yes, so much nicer, so much more subtle. In addition, the relative scarcity and high price of coke lends to its desirability.

There is some question about the addictive effects of coke. Most medical types agree that it is not physically addictive, that is, there are no physical withdrawal symptoms. However, the euphoria and feelings of unlimited energy and extreme power often leads to a heavy psychological addiction with extreme down times when not using.

This postuse depression period makes the heavy user irritable and generally no fun. It has been known to lead to suicide in some really heavy users.

Heavy sniffing of coke can cause perforations of the nasal septum which results in severe nose tissue damage from lack of oxygen.

Coke is an monoamine oxidase inhibitor and one of the most powerful central nervous system stimulants known to mankind. The general rules for MOA inhibitors should be followed when using cocaine. Tolerance does develop with coke to some degree.

COKE SOURCES

The coca plant is actually several different varieties of plant, one of which has less active goodies per area, but has more and larger leaves than its competition. The primary source of cocaine is Peru, where the plants grow in abundance and are still chewed by the fun-loving populace to brighten the humdrum lifestyle a bit.

The main coke plant is a green bush called Erythroxylon Coca. The plant's leaves are harvested by the farmer and his peon buddies and sold to a mobile "lab" truck owner.

The "lab" operator takes the leaves and mixes them with water, benzene, and kerosene. The product is a doughylike paste, called, oddly enough, coca paste. This paste is about 70 per cent cocaine. It takes about 100 pounds of leaves to make one pound of paste.

The paste is sold to a real lab in one of the larger South American cities. Here the paste is processed with sulphuric acid and KMnO and oxalic acid, which precipitates out crystal cocaine.

Occasionally the paste to coke step will be skipped and the coke extracted directly from the leaves with a lime (Na Carbonate) mixture and an organic solvent and treated with sulphuric acid and methanol and extracted with CHCL .

At any rate, the powdered coke is sold for about $1,000 a kilo in South America. The same key is worth about $15,000 – $20,000 (whole) in the States.

STREET COKE

Coke is delivered to the street through (usually) several layers, i.e., it is sold in a key form (pure) and then pounds (minor cutting), say a couple of ounces of milk sugar per pound of coke, to ounces (another cut) to street level buys – grams, spoons, and capsules.

A popular mass book on cocaine emphatically states that because coke goes through so many cuts, street coke is "never more than 5 – 20 per cent pure."

Coke on the West Coast has been averaging about 40 – 60 per cent pure with some GRAMS coming out to 89 – 90 per cent real thing.

Coke is sold in three physical forms: flake, rock, and powder. Most street level sales are in the powder form as this is the most easily diluted. The flakes and rocks are harder to fuck with and are prized by connoisseurs, ALTHOUGH rocks CAN be dissolved and cut and reformed.

Flake is the real coke freak's delight. Flake coke is actually small, fluffy crystals of snow white, sparkly cocaine. It is hard to mix anything with this form and keep the luster and color. Medicinal coke is in flake form.

The price of coke usually runs about $800 – $1,600 per ounce for nice, PURE coke. The pure, medicinal ounce pictured went for $800, although, it would have easily fetched more from record company promo men or others with much money and not too much street sense.

Spoons (a sort of unidentifiable quantity, usually about ¼ – ½ teaspoon) go for $20 – $50 per, and grams hit about $60 – $95 depending on quality and supply. Coke is further broken down into caps of $10 – $20 sizes. This is the least economical format, as one $10 cap is often just one blow.

A pure gram of coke will do about (this is only an estimate, you understand 15 – 20 nice-sized highs.

Street coke is usually snorted (see imbibing section) where it is absorbed by the blood vessels in the mucous membranes and laid out directly to the brain. It can be taken in other methods (shooting gives a real edgy rush) and is often mixed with heroin to form a speedball (sometimes with a psychedelic mixed in).

Shooting coke cuts the total length of the "trip" down, and the user is much more likely to become "addicted" to some degree. The usual needle hassles are, of course, present.

Coke is usually cut with some substance or another to increase the bulk. Common cuts are lactose, which leaves a sweet taste; salt, which is duller and salty tasting; epsom salts; speed; procaine; etc.

Most cuts lose any shininess when crushed into powder; coke crystals do not lose theirs. Procaine and other synthetic local anesthetics produce a much quicker numbing effect than pure coke does, more like a dentist's shot.

If coke is heated over a match some quality judgment is possible. Pure coke burns very clear. Refined coke burns a bit brown and leaves behind a bit of residue. Each cut will leave some sign (salts don't burn, sugars turn to carbon, speed pops as popcorn, procaine causes it to bubble in burning). Of course, the experienced user can often tell by experience how much the drug has been altered.

The cobalt test available in the testing kits is a good indication of the strength of the drug. An intense blue color which forms rapidly after the application of the test substance is a good indication of pure coke.

Coke is often used in conjunction with sex as it stimulates the sexual organs.

Like anything else, coke becomes a problem in too great a quantity. A partial OD of coke produces cold sweat, insomnia, heavy aggression, paranoia, headaches, heavy limbs, etc. Cocaine poisoning can set in with an overdose. The lethal amount of coke is usually between 20 milligrams to 1.3 grams of PURE coke.

Coke is usually snorted with a mini-spoon, chopped with a razor blade for fineness (or passed through a nylon). Often it is snorted through a rolled up dollar bill, although any cokie with real "class" uses nothing less than a $100.

ODs

It is almost impossible to OD on coke, UNLESS it is shot up. Acute cocaine poisoning can then result (one can OD on anything if taken in severe enough quantities or in the wrong way – people still die from salt overdoses every so often) and possibly cardiac arrest. For treatment, see the OD section.

PUSHERS AND USERS

Coke has a definite influence on the user's and even the pusher's lifestyle. Unlike smack, coke pushers tend to indulge in their wares to a great degree. They tend to be very involved in the heavy power-ego-euphoria trip brought on by coke (and also by money, which coke dealers seem to acquire at a prodigious rate) and dress flashy, spend too much in the wrong places, and dig the rep of being a coke dealer.

This game tends to make them quite vulnerable to the authorities, and busts are heavy and common. Coke carries the same weight as heroin in the courts, and they do so like to see dealers go up.

It has been estimated that one out of every ten heavy (ounces-pounds-keys) coke sales is to a narc. This tends to bust a lot of coke dealers and keeps the economy viable by investing great amounts of the government's money in the local street economy of a community.

The big dealers in the coke business are primarily Spanish, or more likely, Cuban. Many of the Cubans who fled to this country to "escape" Castro and who were greeted as heroes (gee, any enemy of Castro's is a friend of mine) were coke dealers trying to escape the Castro regime's crackdown on drugs and criminals in general. The heroic refugees control a major portion of the big coke loads brought into this country from South America and form a sort of Spanish Mafia.

On the street level, coke is dealt by small timers (hippies, college punks, etc.) and on a larger scale by blacks, generally in the ghettos where coke is a consistently excellent seller.

Coke dealers and users, from the top Cubans to the bottom freak, tend to brag too much, like wearing those little gold spoons around their necks or carrying bottles of nose spray everywhere. I mean, the narcs are far from stupid, you know???

GROWTH

Many times the thought of growing coke has crossed the minds of status-quo-minded freaks (how many police know what a coke bush looks like?), but production is nearly nonexistent north of the borders.

The plant grows in the hot climate of the Andes, between 4,000 – 6,000 feet. This climate can be duplicated in greenhouses, but is not found on any great natural basis in the States. (There was a plant in the plant house of San Francisco's Golden Gate Park, but people kept stealing the leaves, so the caretakers were forced to enclose the whole plant in a glass case, at which point, someone stole the entire plant, case and all.)

SYNTHESIS

Possible. Has been published. Difficult, but financially viable with a little work from a topnotch organic chemist. May start to see some in the U.S.

SMALL, FLUFFY CRYSTALS..........................

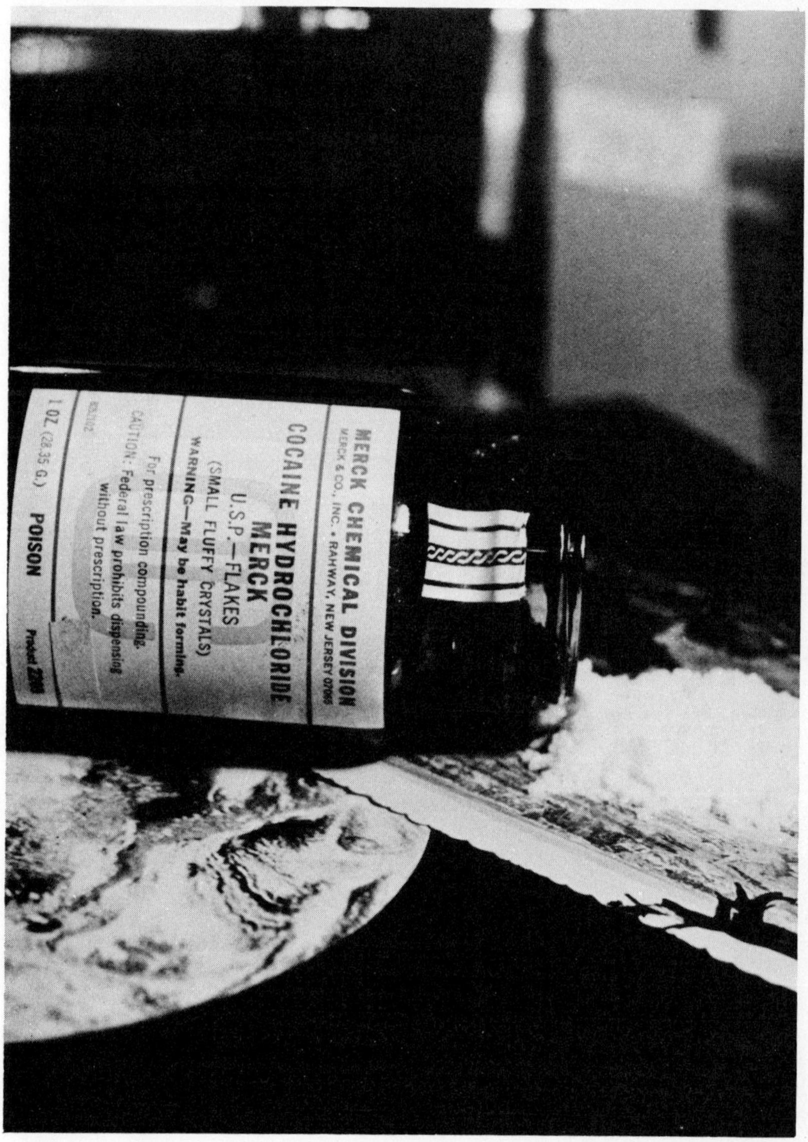

FLUFFING

Fluffing is done to speed, coke, and even heroin to increase the physical bulk and appearance of the drug.

To fluff a drug, it is first chopped crosswise and then back again several times with a sharp razor blade. The chopped drug is then pushed through a fine mesh nylon stocking. This procedure will increase the bulk of a drug by 1½ to 2 times.

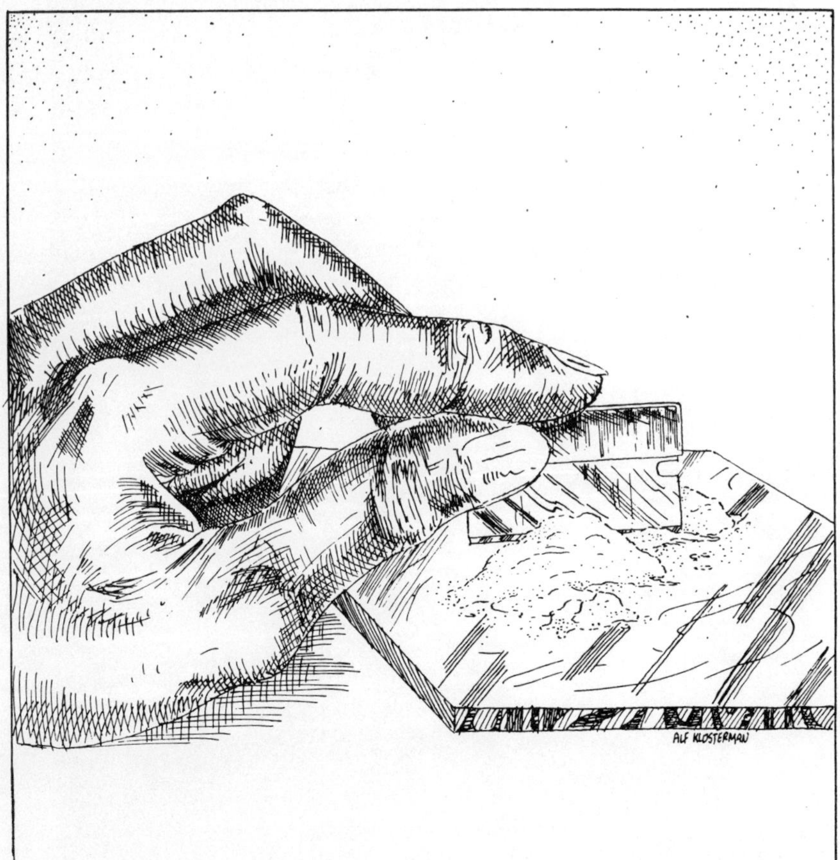

CLASSES OF NARCOTICS

CLASS A — Those drugs which the DEA has classified as addictive and subject to control in manufacture and distribution. They include: codeine, morphine, heroin, cocaine, meperidine, methadone, and all synthetic opiates.

CLASS B — Drugs which the DEA has decided have little or no addictive qualities and which may be prescribed by doctors without filling out a narcotic form. They include: noscapine, nalline, codeine if in quantities smaller than 8 grains per fluid ounce, ethylmorphine in quantities of not more than 1/6 grain per dose, etc.

CLASS M — Special narcotics also considered nonaddictive and able to be prescribed/purchased if not mixed with any other narcotic substance.

CLASS X — Drugs which contain a minute amount of narcotic substance and which can be prescribed without the narcotic order, and occasionally, (notably in the South) can be purchased by signing one's name. They cannot contain (per fluid ounce) more than 1/4 grain of morphine, 1 grain of codeine, or 2 grains of opium. This includes items like paragoric.

CODEINE

A separate alkaloid found in opium,, which is usually extracted by methylizating a morphine base. Its effects mimic those of morphine, but of a milder (figure codeine has about 1/6 to 1/10 the strength of morphine) nature.

Codeine is usually prescribed for the minor pain of headaches, toothaches, and injuries and is felt to be only mildly addictive. The normal prescription dosage ranges from 30 to 60 milligrams.

Codeine, although a class A narcotic (as morphine is), is still found in exempt drugs, notably cough syrup, such as Robitussin AC and other cough fighters with the AC designation.

Codeine may soon be replaced with non-narcotic substitutes in both over-the-counter and prescription drugs.

DET

Diethyltryptamine is a completely synthetic drug similar to DMT. It is easily produced in the lab and the resulting trip is very similar to DMT, although a bit milder and shorter in duration.

DMT

Dimethyltryptamine, or DMT, is an hallucinogen, which is found as a liquid or a colorless crystal. It is a commercial reagent, which used to sell for about $30 a gram from major chemical companies until the FDA and Bureau of Narcotics and Dangerous Drugs clamped the lid on it and required an FDA number to purchase.

DMT is usually smoked on parsley, grass, or tobacco and produces an intense LSD-like trip for about ½ to 2 hours. It has been around as long as LSD and is fairly easy to make. The number of bummers is fairly small, especially for people who relax and don't overdo it the first time.

Organic DMT can be found in such plants as Piptadenia

and Banisteriopsis, and other DMT derivatives can still be purchased on the open market (See legal highs section).

DOB

A relatively new addition to the underground market DOB (4-Bromo-2, 5-Dimethoxyphenylisopropylamine) was first synthesized in 1970. It is an amphetamine based drug very close to STP (the 4 methoxy group of STP [DOM] is replaced with a bromine atom) in chemical make up.

DOB seems to bring on a high which resembles that of MDA, with increased physical and intellectual stimulation, but lacking the visual distortions present in an LSD or STP trip.

The "usual" DOB tripper seems to experience a closeness with his environment and a definite increase in his attention levels. This may lead to the proverbial long term inspection of leaves or other objects close at hand as well as a feeling of really "understanding" things/people. The trip intensifications are not unlike those brought about by mescaline, a fact which will, no doubt, lead to DOB winding up as "mescaline" in the street...........

The intensity of the trip seems to increase with the amount, up to a leveling off point occurring around 2 mills. The average hit of DOB is about 1 milligram.

DOB is fairly easy and inexpensive to make and is already showing up in testing centers across the country under various pseudonyms.

HASHISH

The pure resinous exudate of the female marijuana plant. It is usually seen in the form of brown lumps, after hardening with exposure to the air. Hash is the most potent form of marijuana available, with the exception of hash oils.

In India, hash is known as charas and usually smoked, while in Africa it is often eaten. The smoker experiences a less potent trip as he can regulate his intake with the degree of the stone, while the eater must suffer the full dose. The final stage of a hash "OD" is a deep comalike sleep which can last for 18 hours.

There is only a slight degree of tolerance buildup in hash, much of which may be attributed to the user learning to control his trip to a greater degree.

Hash costs between $60 and $100 an ounce in the U.S. and tends to last about the same length of time as a pound of marijuana.

Heavy concentrations of THC (such as that found in good hash) give rise to similar trips as mescaline or even LSD, although there is no chemical resemblance between the drugs. There is no indole ring or nitrogen in its structure, and researchers are a bit unsure as to what makes the drug act this way. As with grass, there is a dilation of the blood vessels when smoking hash. This accounts for the reddening of the eyes. Any THC product releases insulin into the blood, causing the body to consume blood sugar and can produce a craving for sweets.

Most Middle East hash that reaches the U.S. is between 5 - 12 per cent THC. Grass that contains 1 - 4 per cent is usually considered heavy dope, normal American smoking weed checks in at about 1 per cent.

A sometimes rule of thumb for hash is: the darker the hash, the more potent it is likely to be. Indian hash is darker and harder than American or Mexican and usually about four - six times as strong. Moroccan and African can get into near black and are usually quite potent, while Lebanese comes in a blond shade that is nice, but generally less potent. Of course, each country has its own various grades of hash, and this rule of thumb is not perfect, but it is generally true.

Hash, although chemically identical to the active ingredient in marijuana, produces a different high. It is generally (although this is not true in heavy doses) less sedative and more hallucinogenic.

Ancient warriors (the Zarathustrians, no less) chewed hash before going into battle to screw up their courage. The term "assassin" may have come from the term hashish.

Hashish used to enjoy a medical reputation as a good anesthetic as it is safer and better than morphine or any other modern day anesthetic, but when the big hemp scare started coming down, it was no longer medically employed.

VARIETIES

Nepalese hash, a dark brown-black variety is one example of a consistently strong, good hash. The common packaging methods for Nepalese is in the form of temple balls, so named for their frequent presence at Buddhist rites. They are hand rolled, with the darker varieties usually having a touch of opium added to round out the high.

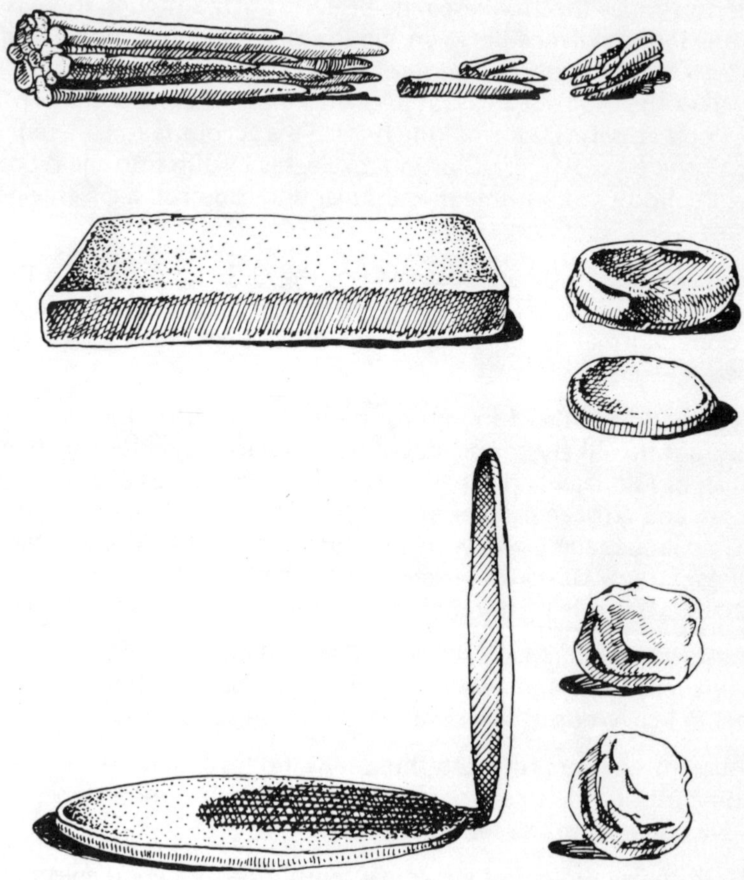

Various formats of imported hash: (upper) "fingers" – Nepal; (middle upper) "brick" – Morocco; (lower left) "surfboards" – Afghanistan (middle right) "patties" – Afghanistan, (lower right) "temple balls" – Nepal.

Nepalese also comes in "fingers", a somewhat coarser variety than the temple balls, but still nice.

Pakistan mass-produces fairly high quality hash, usually the color of dark leather. Pakistan hash comes in several grades, the better ones usually have the gold seal of the Frontier Constabulary, a "police" organization in the rugged Pakistan territories where the hash originates.

Pakistan is not to be sneezed at, but, with the exception of the very top grades, usually lacks just a bit over the Nepalese, and is not quite as good a seller.

Lebanese hash does not seem to be in the heaviest stone class, but the finer grades are a real connoisseur's treat, imparting a nice easy head high. The poorer grades are likely to be a bit harsh.

Afghanistan hash tends to lack the stickiness of the other varieties and often uses animal fat to bind the chips together. This gives it a definite "earthy" odor which distinguishes it from all others. Afghanistani is usually quite potent hash and commands a fairly high price.

PRICE

Hash, like any other drug, commands what price it can get. That is to say, when grass is lush and available, hash prices seem to drop, and the poorer qualities have a hard time selling at all. When grass becomes scarce, hash prices tend to rise.

The average price for a good ounce of hash is $70 - $100 with individual grams going for $5 - $10.

USING

Hash is usually smoked in a small pipe (while resting on a screen) or mixed with tobacco in a cigarette or added to a joint. However, real connoisseurs normally employ a water pipe, which filters it out a bit and cools down the smoke, or a chillum (See instructions).

GETTING

Hash can be gathered from your crop by rubbing the flowers between your hands or beating them against a piece of scrap leather. The collected resin is the hash.

CHILLUM

The chillum is an ancient device designed to amplify the high produced by hash smoking. It is a straight clay pipe which narrows down to end in a small opening.

The chillum consists of three pieces: the chillum, or pipe; the gehee, a small irregularly shaped stone, which fits about 1/3 of the way down the chillum and lodges there (the hash is placed on the stone, and the smoke escapes around it); the sophee, a damp rag, which is folded over the business end of the chillum to filter and cool the smoke.

There is a certain, deft technique required in preparing a chillum, but the results are superb.

1. Take a lump of hash (anywhere from ¼ to 1 gram) and heat it by crossing two lit matches and placing the hash on the "Y" of the cross. A quick heating will do, just enough to make the hash crumble when touched.

2. Take an equal amount of tobacco (or grass, if you're not into tobacco) and mix it with the hash. The moisture from the tobacco will blend the two just right — mash them together into one lump.

3. Place the hash/tobacco in the chillum on top of the rock. Place the damp cloth over the opening in the narrow end of the chillum.

4. Now, lay the chillum between the middle three fingers of your left hand to form a seal as shown. Wrap the other hand around it (usually in between the little finger and the fourth finger) to make an airtight seal, except for a small hole.

5. Light the hash and suck the joyous gases through the small hole in your fingers. The object here is not to hold it in your lungs as one might with grass or a normal hash pipe, but rather to hyperventilate the gases into your lungs by inhaling deeply, immediately exhaling, and repeating the process a couple of more times without a break.

This technique gives a different stone than a normal hash pipe. You get off as well, if not better, and the tobacco gives a little boost to the THC, the whole mess producing a nice head stone with tobacco rushes up and down the spine.

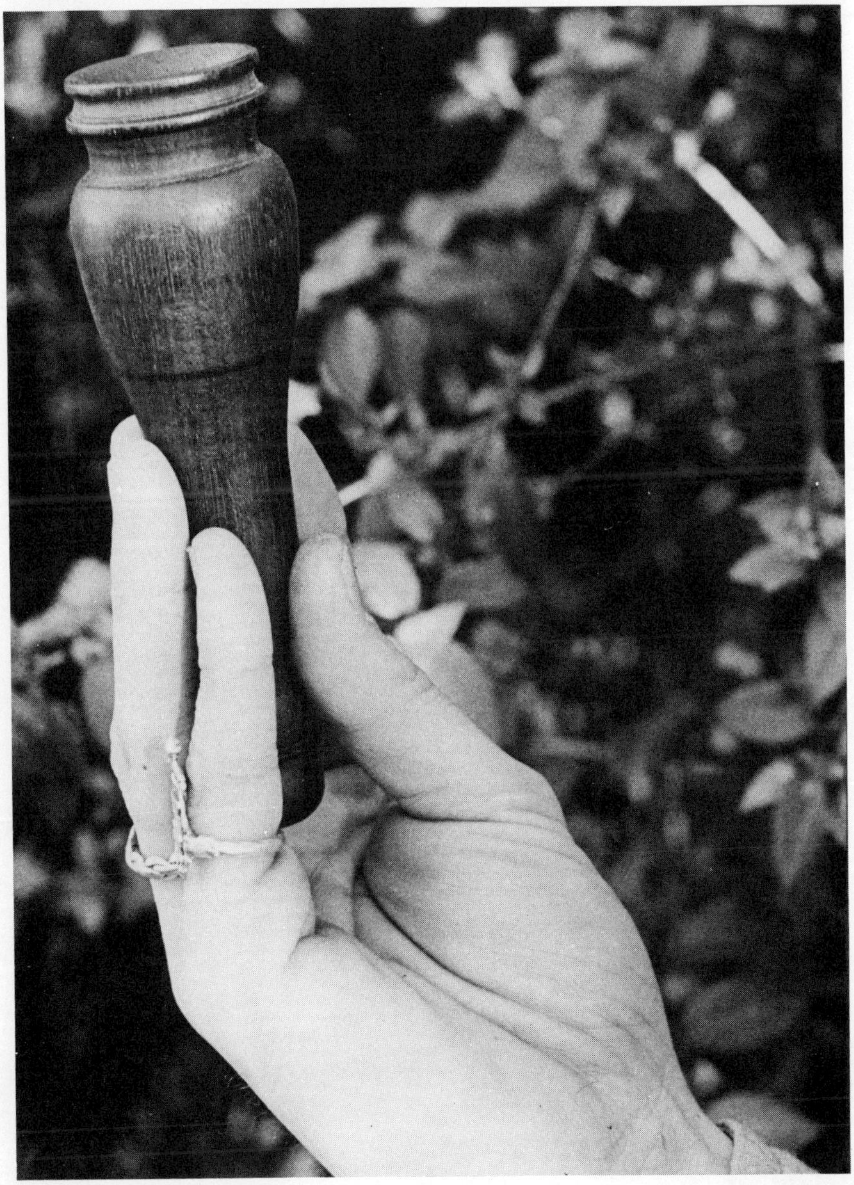

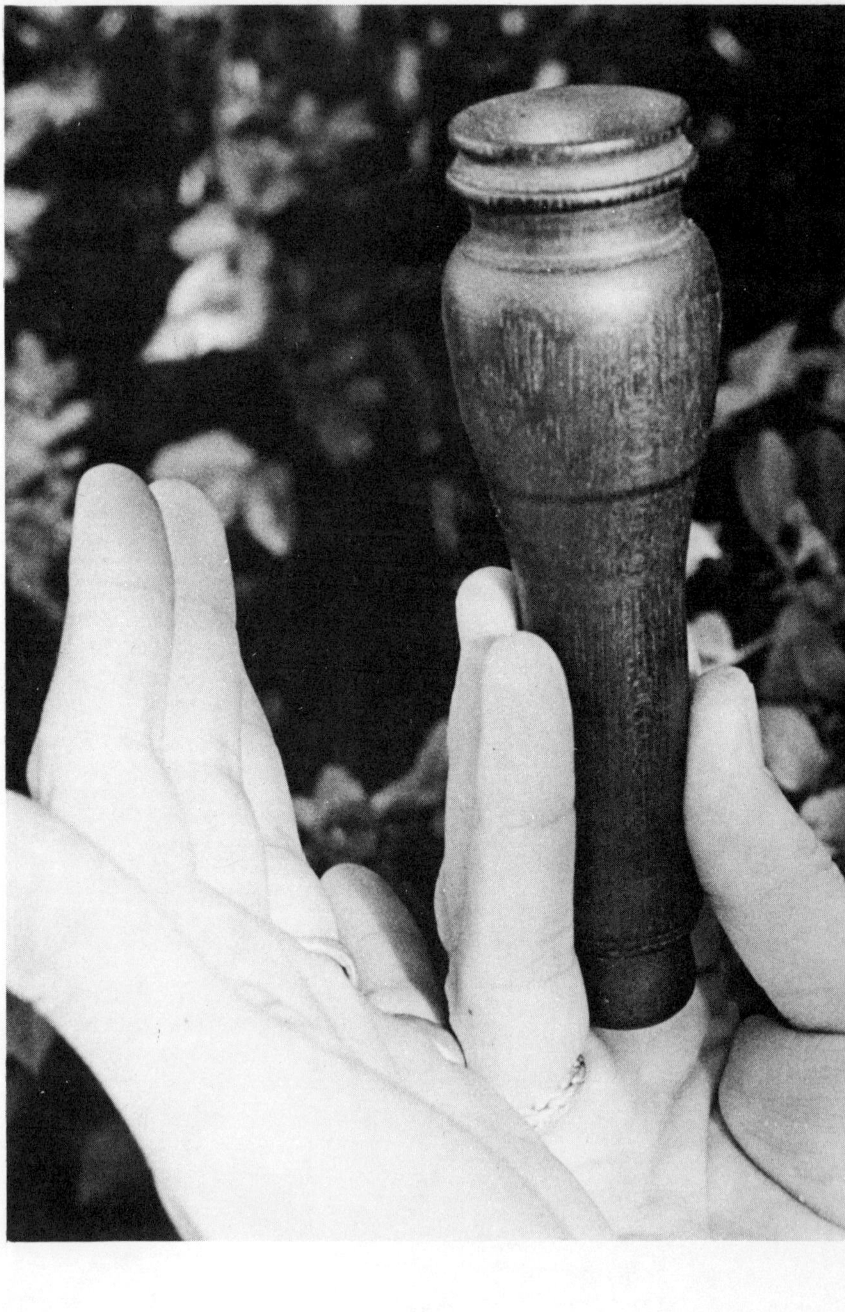

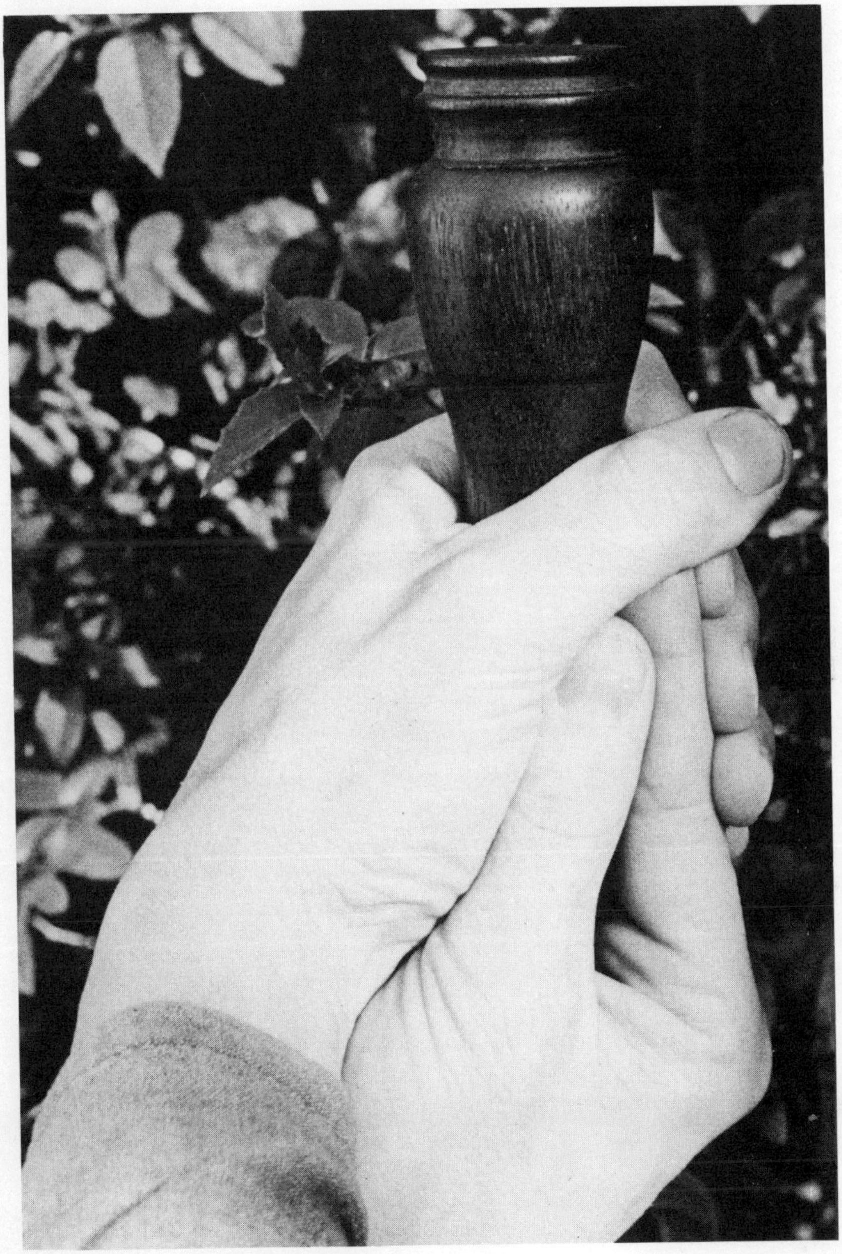

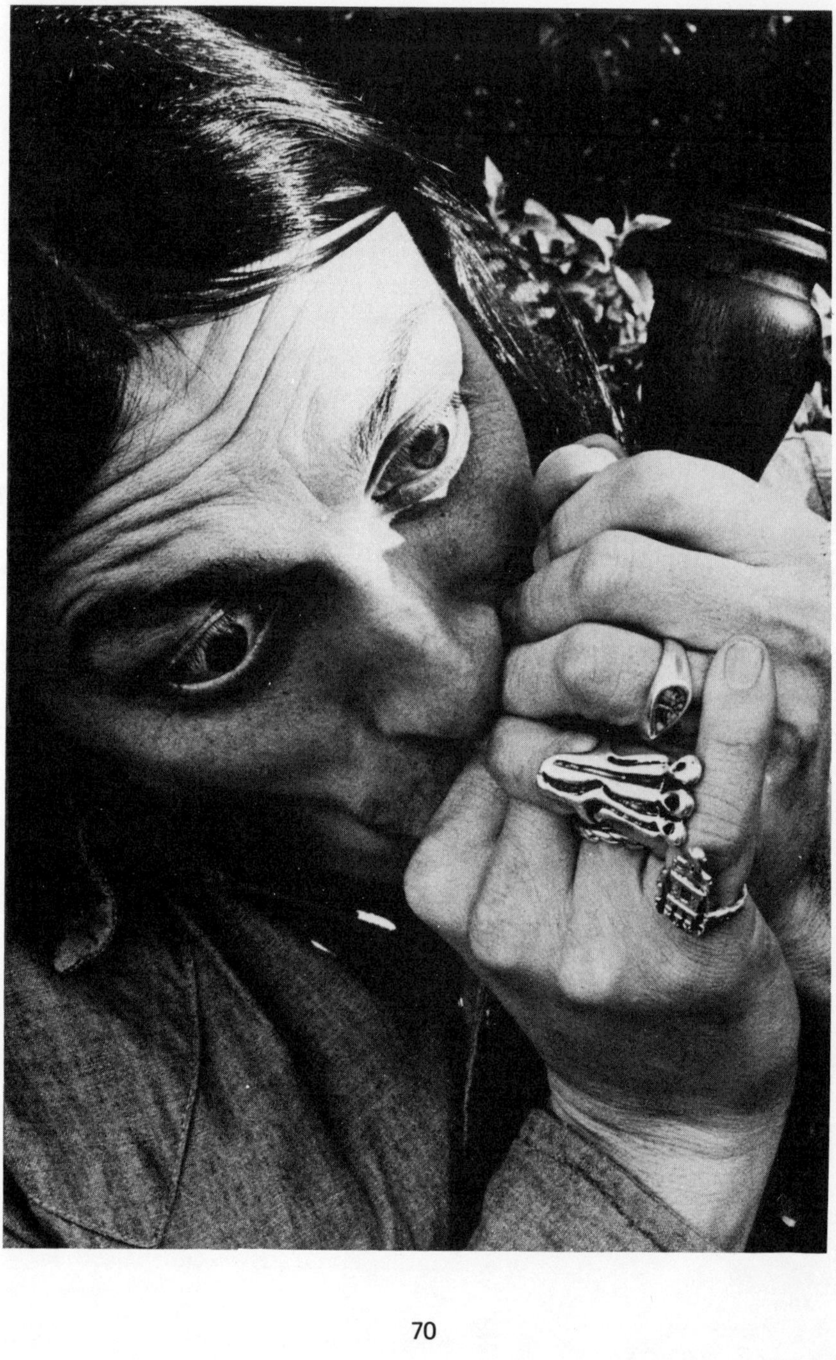

HOME HASH MANUFACTURE

There are several "formulas" for making your own hash. These formulas involve cutting the resin out of grass and mixing it with a thickener, such as finely ground "good" grass or ashes. Of course, this is not really hash, but can give a similar effect (but not exactly the same as real hash) when smoked. The problem with this idea is, of course, when you've lifted the resin out of the grass, don't expect to sell the grass any more. As it is usually easier to use/dispose of grass than hash the economics of this operation make little sense.

The one possible exception to this rule is when you have a large quantity of poor quality grass. You can often extract the resin that is available and concentrate it into "hash." To do this, simply follow the recipe included for resin extraction and mix the product with some powdered top-quality grass as shown in the hash oil section.

HASH AND GRASS OILS

Marijuana extracts have been utilized in medicine since the early 1800s, but curiously enough, have just found their way into the hip scene within the last few years.

In the 1960s, scientists first synthesized THC (tetrahydrocannabinol). Underground chemists tried to make it feasible for the hip market but the cost still remains a prohibitive barrier to underground manufacture.

The first hash oil known to hit the market was in 1970 and was called "the one" and made by a group called the "Cosmic Traveller." Small vials containing about five grams sold for about $150 complete with two small pyrex ONE pipes and a xerox copy of instructions to get the whole thing off the ground.

The oil was a dirty, dark chocolate in color and was a thick goo in consistency. The oil was a pure, organic extract of marijuana with a bit of ground-up weed added to bring it down to smoking consistency. It seemed to be an alcohol cut of top mexi-weed and contained about 13 per cent THC. (Normal grass contains less than 1 per cent. The top weed used in government experiments runs 4 per cent and most volunteers rate it as the best they have ever had. Good hash ranges from 8 - 14 per cent THC.)

Some of ONE appeared about September 1971 and sold for $125 - $130 for a five gram vial, with a bit bigger ONE pipe. It was less potent than the first ONE, and seemed to have a bit more ground-

(continued on p. 77)

OIL MANUFACTURE NO. 1

It is possible to extract the active oil from marijuana. This THC can be stored in the liquid form (for ease in storage or hiding) and then reapplied to parsley, hops, etc. for a true grass potency.

Fifty pounds of grass will produce about one — two pounds of resin which can then be redissolved and reapplied or sold directly as THC.

To remove the THC from grass or hash, you must cover it with a suitable solvent (isopropyl alcohol, benzene, methanol will all work) and all soaked on LOW heat for about 12 hours. More solvent must be added to combat evaporation.

Filter the solvent and repeat for another 12 hours.

Evaporate the combined solvent extracts until a syrupy resin is obtained or until it solidifies.

Repeat this process on the grass until a quick smoke shows that all the THC has been removed.

HASH AND GRASS OIL MANUFACTURE NO. 2

Reduce the substance to a powder by use of a blender and/or mortar and pestle. Now weigh the powdered mixture. Wash the material in warm water several times, straining the water and throwing it out until the wash is clear.

Add water to an amount of sodium carbonate equal to ½ the weight of your starting materials. Add the powdered hash or grass to this mixture, adding more water if necessary to cover the material.

On LOW heat (a pilot light is perfect) let this mixture "work" for 48 hours.

Now strain the mixture through a cloth filter, squeezing the water out. Dry the solid material and throw away the liquid.

Wet the material with ethyl alcohol until damp and place in a tightly closed jar for six hours. Add alcohol, if necessary, to maintain dampness.

Place the material in a separatory funnel, with a small piece of cotton in the drain tube. Pack the material in to maximum tightness.

Saturate the material with ethyl alcohol until a thin liquid layer remains on top. Close the petcock and seal the top for 48 hours.

After this time, open the petcock and let the liquid drip out into an open container. Add more ethyl alcohol to again soak the material fully.

After approximately one quart of alcohol has been used for every kilo of raw materials, drop a few drops of liquid into a test tube of water and watch for the appearance of an oily extract to appear. When this oily extract/precipitate no longer appears, the removal of the active constituents is complete.

Now make a solution of suspended calcium hydroxide in water by adding one ounce of calcium hydroxide for every one pound of raw material. Add the chemical to water and shake until it is completely suspended in solution. Use as much water as necessary.

Add the alcohol/THC mixture to the calcium hydroxide solution and shake well. Filter the mixture through a cheese cloth, squeeze it dry, and throw away the solids.

Now, add a small bit of sulfuric acid to the mixture to make any excess calcium hydroxide drop out of solution. Add some animal charcoal to the mixture and filter through the cheese cloth again. By evaporation or distillation, remove most of the alcohol. The mixture should have the consistency of thin syrup.

Weigh the remainder and add twice its weight in water. Shake and let the rest of the alcohol evaportae. Now, mix with water again and separate the two layers with the separatory funnel, throwing away the water. You should continue washing and separating until the water layer tests out to a neutral ph (7).

After the final evaporation, place the oil in a tightly closed container.

OIL MANUFACTURE NUMERO THREE

While similar in design to number one, this method is probably the most universal and may, in fact, be the best.

With grass, follow the smashing/crunching processes already described. Then, heat in a low (around 250) oven for 10 minutes. With hash, heat a bit first and then grind into fine powder.

Now the crushed cannabis is boiled in a THC soluble solvent. This is normally methanol, although pure grain alcohol (ethanol) will work as well, if not better.

You must realize that boiling any alcohol-or ether-based solvent releases dangerous fumes which will injure one if inhaled and may explode if exposed to any flame. For this reason, you must always boil in a semi-closed system, or at least, under a well-ventilated lab hood. Always use an electric stove/hotplate or even better, a lab reflux.

The refluxing is done by placing the cannabis/solvent mixture (amounts are not critical — just enough to cover all the material) in a flask in a water bath (to keep the temperature below 100 degrees C) and place on the electric heater.

It is possible to create a home-brew system by utilizing pots, plastic bags, and a steel lid containing ice for the condenser, but I prefer to use a flask and a commercial lab condenser.

Heat the mixture for a couple of hours, allowing the solvent to drip back into the flask after condensing. After this step is completed place all the solvent/oil mixture in another flask and put the soggy cannabis material in a filter paper-lined funnel leading into the flask. Arrange the condenser so you can boil (in the water bath again) the oil/solvent and allow it to condense and drip down through the soggy cannabis material, much as a coffee pot drips the liquid back through the grounds to get all the good stuff. . .After the drops become clear, you can figure all the oil has been extracted from the grass.

At this point in time, so to speak, you must get rid of the solvent. This is accomplished by boiling the solvent and oil in the water bath (methanol or ethanol will vaporize at about 94 degrees centigrade) until only the oil remains. Be sure to use a damn good ventilating hood, or better yet, condense the solvent and reuse it in your next science fair project. The remaining syrup is the THC-laden oil minus all solvent.

NOW WHAT?

Once you have your hash or grass oil there are several things you can do with it to improve or at least change its effects:

PURIFICATION

It is possible to further purify the oil by a petroleum ether extraction (ED. NOTE: regular ether and petroleum ether are two different animals and CANNOT be substituted for each other.). This method will decrease the total amount of oil, but will increase the potency of the remainder.

Mix the oil with alcohol at a 1 (oil) to 5 (alcohol) ratio and then mix the results with a like volume of water. Place this mixture in an open flask or stirring jar and place on a magnetic stirrer or hand stir with much vigor, for several minutes.

Mix the total mixture with a volume of petroleum ether of a volume equaling one half of everything else and restir (again, preferably with a mag stirrer) for 10 minutes.

Now place in a separatory funnel (a glass funnel with a tube and petcock extending from its base to control the flow of the liquid). Three distinct layers will appear after 20 minutes or so: the bottom will be alcohol and various impurities, the middle will be ether, and the top will be a combination of ether and the good stuff. Drain off all but the top layer. Take this layer and add more petroleum ether, restir, let sit, reseparate, once again saving only the top layer. When this is completed the ether should remain clear, signifying that all impurities have been removed.

Next place the ether oil mixture in a flask which is placed in the proverbial water bath and heat (again only on a lab reflux or electric stove) to 140 degrees F. At this point, the ether will boil off (the temperature will stabilize here until the ether is boiled off). When you feel it has all boiled away you can raise the temperature of the water for a few minutes to make sure all the alcohol is also gone. The THC oil will not boil off at this temperature.

INCREASING THE STRENGTH

There is a process which you can perform on the cleaned oil which will increase its potency without losing much quantity.

All grass/hash oils contain a certain percentage of THC (depending on level of purification and quality of the starting material) and a number of related but as far we as are concerned, inert, substances which (such as cannabidiol) can be converted into active THC. This process will also help raise the quality of the existing THC to a more digestable level.

Dissolve the oil in straight methanol at a 1 (oil) to 10 (methanol) ratio. Now CAREFULLY add a drop of CONCENTRATED sulfuric acid for every gram of oil in the mixture. Once again I must reiterate, do not work with such things as sulfuric acid without the proper knowledge and safety equipment (glasses, gloves, lab apron, etc.).

Reflux in a boiling pot for a couple of hours and then let cool and pour into an equal volume of water. Now mix with a like volume of petroleum ether and use a sep funnel to save only the ether/oil layer.

Mix the ether with 5 times its volume of water, stir for a time, pour into the sep funnel, and discard the water layer.

Pour the ether layer into a solution of water and bicarbonate of soda (made from 1 part soda to 20 parts water). Stir, separate the layers, and save the ether/oil layer.

Mix with pure water and separate, twice. Place the final ether solution *in a flask and boil the ether off (again, at about 140 degrese F). The remainder is heavy duty oil. . .*

TRICKS AND QUIRKS

There are several things you can do with your oil besides the obvious; it can be turned into "THC pills" by combining the oil with the same quantity of butter and then mixing both with some inert filler such as Similac, flour, etc., and then capping in a large capsule.

This method allows a higher quantity of THC to enter the bloodstream than consuming the straight oil does.

Dark oil may be transmuted into so-called, "honey oil," which tends to taste a bit better and smoke a trifle cleaner, but really does not get one off to any greater degree, by weighing the oil and combining it with a solution of pure methanol of at least 12 times the oil's volume and then adding a quantity of activated charcoal granules roughly equal to the weight of the starting oil. Now mix well and filter through filter paper.

Evaporate the methanol off and the honey oil will remain.

If you have extracted the oil from medium or poor quality grass and wish to make "hash" from your oil, you can mix it with finely powdered, top-quality grass (a mortar and pestle, rolling pin, or good blender will do the trick) until the appearance and potency of hash is attained.

It often helps if you heat the grass in a LOW oven for 20 minutes prior to the mix job. Figure about 13 per cent oil to 77 per cent grass for a passable street quality hash, up to/through a 40/60 mixture for hash that will contact stone the people in the next house. . .

(continued from p. 71)
up grass in it.

BLACK OIL surfaced in California in early January 1972. It was a dark black, thin fluid made from grass, but did not appear to have been mixed with powdered weed and hence, was runnier. It seemed to be an alcohol tincture and was probably double cut with ether. It was harsh on the ol' throat, but was fairly potent.

The best quality oil is not made from grass, but rather from hash. It is also called RED OIL from the work done in the 1940s by Dr. Adams. In mid-1971 this oil first appeared in the form of a gooey, honey-colored preparation. It was supposedly extracted from a Lebanese hash base and probably fractionally distilled to get the THC out from the other active isomers in the plant.

It had a very low boiling point and had to be stored in a cool, dark place. A gram of real hash oil went for as much as $50 - $60. It could have run as high as 18 - 20 per cent THC.

Any OIL can be eaten, but the OD is a great risk. When smoking oils one should proceed with much caution and take in less than your hash experience tells you you should be taking in.

All oils cannot be burned directly but must be vaporized by heating them from underneath in a pyrex pipe. You put a tiny bit of oil on the inside of the pipe and then hold it in the flame of a match (not too good) or gas or alcohol burner (better) for a couple of seconds. You will hear it sizzle and vapors will rise as it begins to vaporize, at this point one should take VERY VERY gently (or experienced hash smokers will feel themselves coughing like first timers). About two hits should do you up for an hour — three definitely.

I am listing several methods for hash and grass oil extraction. Any of these will work. As usual, the more difficult systems will have the best yield.

It is possible to make the oil for the simple joy of it; or because you want to make "hash," or "THC Pills"; or because you want to extract the resins, make the THC stronger, and reapply it to the original grass.

Occasionally someone will extract the oil from grass in another country (now, Mexico does come to mind), hide the comparable small quantity of oil, smuggle it into the States, and then reapply it to some vegetarianlike substance and sell it as good weed.

HEROIN

Heroin comes from a German word meaning large or powerful,

an apt description. It is a semisynthetic derivative of morphine, made by treating morphine with acetic anhydride. Pure heroin is a white crystalline (except Mexican, which is brown) powder with a slight bitter taste.

Heroin was originally discovered and put to use as a treatment for morphine addiction. In the purest sense, this treatment was quite successful, most morphine addicts soon ended their problem with morphine.

It was twelve long years before the various people in positions of responsible authority noticed the reformed morphine addicts were acting strangely when they couldn't get any heroin...

It was also sold over the counter as a sure-fire cure for coughing, depression, and a number of other sicknesses, real or imagined. Heroin is about 20 - 25 times as potent as morphine and about four times more addictive.

Heroin is so potent that it can survive a radical number of cuts and still be salable, hence, it is an ideal dealer's drug. The top men buy pure pounds, hit them with Epsom salts, quinine, etc., and sell fairly pure ounces which are hit again and sold as potent quarters, hit again and sold as nice spoons, hit again and sold as average dime bags, hit again and sold as mild capsules for $1 - $3. Most street bags are from 1½ per cent to 3 per cent pure H.

This makes a situation where just about anybody with a little capital can make money and still support a habit. Most users eventually get into one level of dealing or another to support the trip.

Most of the world's supply of heroin comes from the Eastern countries where the magic poppy grows. It is scraped as residue from the poppy and boiled into opium, cut into morphine base by the village "collector," smuggled out of the area (often into Marseilles), cut into heroin (which is the least bulky and most expensive form — about half the bulk of powdered morphine) and smuggled into the United States, usually by "organized" crime, at one level of "organization" or another.

One kilo of opium seeds in Turkey sells for about $40 and one kilo of smack sells for about $45,000 in the U.S.

As a general rule, West Coast smack is less potent than that of the East Coast, possibly due to the fact that most "pure" reaches the U.S. through an East Coast port and must travel through a number of hands before arriving in California. Of course, the East Coast has a much higher number of junkies than the West.

Smack is a much different scene than the other drugs (psychedel-

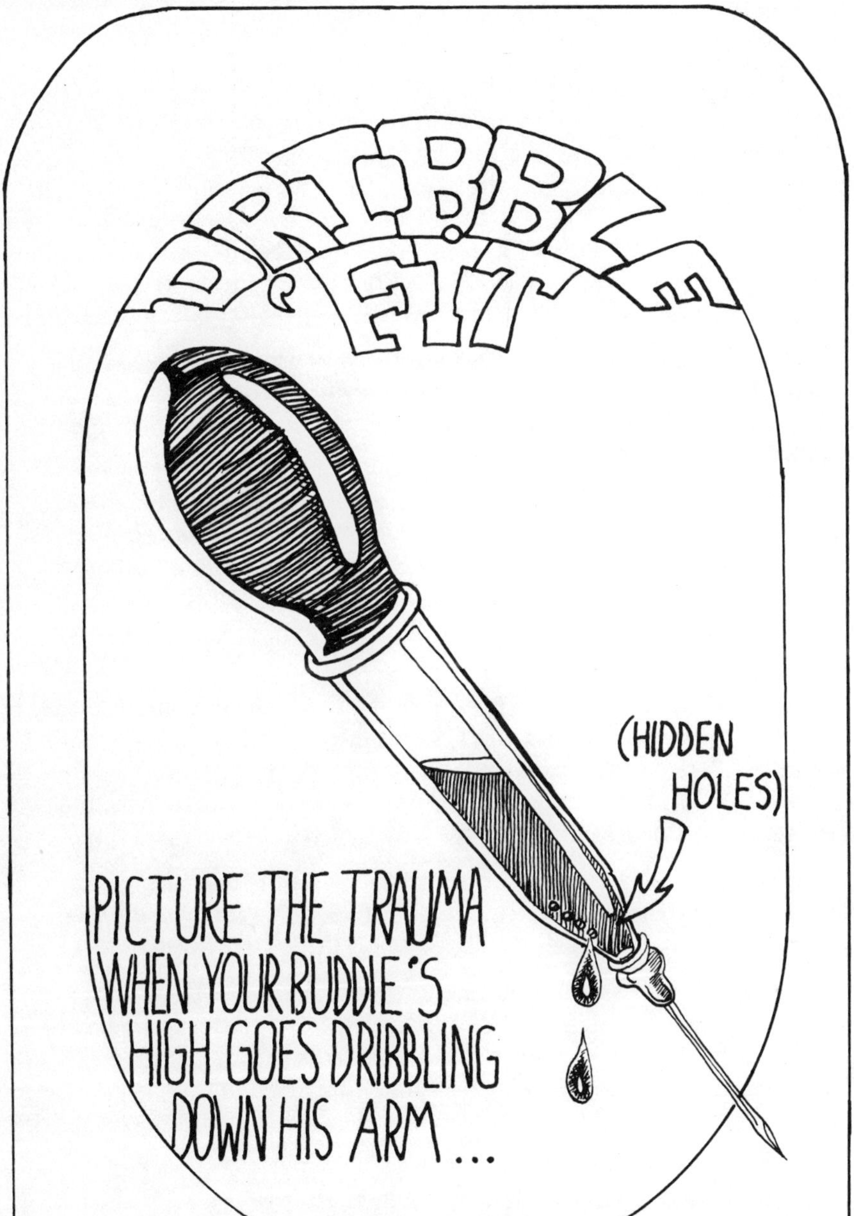
DRIBBLE FIT
(HIDDEN HOLES)
PICTURE THE TRAUMA WHEN YOUR BUDDIE'S HIGH GOES DRIBBLING DOWN HIS ARM . . .

ics, grass, uppers, etc.). Normally, the same people are not involved with both sets of drugs, the grass psychedelic culture tends to frown on smack users.

There are exceptions to this rule. For a time in the early 70s, smack began rearing its ugly head in the middle class kid's repertoire at an increasing frequency. Much of this was due to the misleading drug information pushed on the public by the press and government. I mean, if they claim that grass is all that bad, why believe them when they knock heroin? With this reasoning, a number of grassers migrate into heroin every time a series of crackdowns by the ever-faithful government dries up the grass supply.

Heroin can be sniffed or injected. Many users start out with a "taste" by sniffing and gradually move on to injecting as they use larger amounts. Injecting loses less of the potency and makes the quantity go further.

Popping or muscular injections can take place anywhere in the body. Mainlining, or intravenously injecting, is the preferred form. It produces an initial flash of high intensity (much like an orgasm) lacking in either sniffing or popping and leaves the drug in its highest potency.

The addict will often begin hitting in the main arm vein, near the inside of the elbow, as it is easy to find and close to the surface. As he uses more and more smack, he usually switches to other veins, due to the "tracks" or scars that develop, making it obvious to the casual observer what is going on, as well as hardening the vein, making a successful hit nearly impossible.

Long-time addicts get into a constant search-for-a-virgin-vein hassle and hit themselves on the legs, between the toes, inside the thighs, the jugular veins, and occasionally, under the tongue.

Heroin is prepared by mixing with a small quantity of water. Pure heroin will dissolve at this point, but street heroin must be heated to dissolve properly. This is often done in a bottle cap by a match. The addict then ties off a vein, by tying a tourniquet on the area (or whatever) above the vein with a belt or, as is preferred, a surgical rubber tube.

The melted/dissolved smack is drawn up into the user's outfit (or "fit"); a syringe made from an eye dropper with a hypodermic needle on one end and the rubber bulb from a baby's pacifier on the other. This is used, instead of a normal medical syringe, because it gives the user better control over the valuable liquid in the tube.

The needle is inserted into a vein and the rubber bulb relaxed to get a "flag", or bit of red blood in the solution, indicating a vein has been struck. The bulb is then pressed and the liquid rushes into the user. Some addicts will resuck as much of the liquid (and of course, blood and other bodily fluids) back into the fit and reshoot in an attempt to relive the initial slash several times.

Heroin produces a stupor-state of incredible dullness to any outside stimuli – the user has no or little interest in sex, food, pain, moving, or other red-blooded American pastimes. Instead, he just wants to lie there in his pure bliss and ignore the world for several hours. Most addicts are seeking heavy escape (many times a justifiable escape, it may be noted) from their lifestyle. It is an easy way to reach the superlative. You don't need fancy cars, loads of money, or nice-looking girls to live the American dream – just a quick fix.

This pastime "tripping" gradually (depending on the strength and number of doses) changes into a situation where the addict feels very uncomfortable without heroin. He begins to exhibit signs of a severe cold (runny nose, chills, irritability, stomach upset) when he is between hits.

This worsens into severe withdrawal symptoms as the user becomes more and more hooked. He must keep a new shot every few hours just to function normally. The main thing on the user's mind becomes how to get enough smack to get "straight."

One of the sad parts of this dilemma is the fact that he is using it more and enjoying it less – the high is not nearly so intense as his tolerance builds up. He needs larger and larger doses just to keep moving.

Chronic users tend to commit themselves for detoxification in various hospitals or in Lexington when their tolerance level gets too high. This kicking process takes about three weeks and then they are clean. Many start shooting again right away, but they get by with smaller doses.

Heroin in itself is not physiologically harmful. It is the whole lifestyle that leads to trouble. Malnutrition, hepatitis from "borrowing" fits, bronchitis, collapsed veins, abscesses and other malfunctions are common symptoms of the smack user.

Persons who don't believe that heroin addiction is really a severe, physical thing should realize that a typical New York junkie must spend about $10,000 a year on his habit. This means that he must steal between $40,000 and $50,000 worth of goods to resell for the drug money. Now that takes some heavy motivation.

Smack addiction is no fun to kick, but in reality, it is far less

(continued on p. 87)

Law and order. Order and law. It never ceases to amaze me how we can have so much rhetoric on this particular subject and so little action.

I mean, have you tried to take an evening walk in any major American city of late? Who says the last frontier is dead? Got a spirit of adventure or an unmitigated blood lust? Just take a stroll down Fourth Street, or Fillmore, or Woodward, or, or, or. . .

So what's to be done about this shitty situation? Do we violate the law ourselves and carry .357 magnums, rent police dogs, and go on the buddy system? Or do we each carry a police whistle, as suggested by a New York Congressman, to blow upon when danger threatens?

You gotta admit, this last suggestion conjures up all sorts of interesting pictures? You, blowing feverishly on your Edward Koch police whistle while surrounded by 14 delirium-eyed, DTed, half-naked black junkies armed with straight razors, butcher knives, and assorted bottles and car antennas, waiting for the forces of law and order to respond to your whistled asylum. . .and waiting. . .and waiting. . .and waiting. . .

So we must examine the roots of crime and social degeneration. Is it class-conscious blacks springing forth from the ghettos to take their rightful place in the American dream? Is it armed revolutionaries attacking the merits of high living to redistribute the wealth? (An interesting interjection here is when the confirmed "revolutionary" Stephanie Kline decided her group of "revolutionaries" needed to raise some money to help the "cause" as well as distribute the corporate wealth, a la Robin Hood, she and her friends robbed, now get this; do they attack ITT, Standard Oil, the Pentagon? No. . .they hit upon the CO-OP market. . .) Is the Mafia behind street crime? No, oddly enough the major percentage of muggings, robberies, and burglaries are all committed by one low life creature known as the junkie.

Son-of-a-bitching junkies are everywhere like roaches in the ghetto. They are crawling up fire escapes, smashing windows, hitting people on the head, and ODing in the alleys. A more disagreeable bunch you could not find than stinking, slit-your-brother's-throat-for-a-dime-bag junkies.

Now, here we should make a distinction. I'm not talking about the evils of heroin. Heroin is just a little white, passive powder. Dig it, it never attached anyone and forced itself upon him against his will. Nor is it injected into people by the police in heavy questioning sessions or forced on little kids in school yards by the neighborhood pusher.

No, $C_{17}H_{17}NO(C_2H_3)_2$ is just the final product of the poppy flower, put here on God's green earth for some concrete reason in the general scheme of things. By itself it poses no threat to anyone.

There is just one path to attaining junkiehood; get some smack and use it, and then get some more and use that, and get some, etc., etc., over a fair period of time.

Now, this takes some real doing. Ths shit is hard to find, expensive, tends to make one sick the first few times, and difficult to take. Besides which, the junkie-to-be knows just what he is getting himself into. No one ever did up some smack in a drunken fit and became hooked the next afternoon. No, it takes some real effort.

Now, you out there who fancy yourself social scientists of one level or another, can blame any number of alienating factors, from housing to lack of education, to society in general, for this occurrence. I don't know, maybe you're right, but the point is the junkie is taking the smack because he wants to, knowing full well what he is getting into. Pity for the junkie is like cultivating rats for pets. Don't go to sleep around them.

If the junkie gets "hooked" due to some great personal tragedy, or truly without realizing what has happened, he can always stop. Yes, that's right. He can just stop. A few days of sickness (rough, but not like having both legs smashed between car bumpers or anything) and bingo, he's no longer a junkie. Now maybe he doesn't have the will power to stop. Fine, there are any number of organizations which will help him stop in any fashion he chooses, up to, and including, supporting him and his dependents during the process, and substituting other drugs for the joys of heroin.

How many other "diseases" have those kinds of facilities available for the average guy on the street?

No, the junkie is a dirty low life rat who steals from his friends and neighbors in any way he can to support an enjoyable habit which he is cultivating. There is nothing heroic or even pitiful about this — just sickening.

So what do we do? Keep electing politicians who talk about the dope "problem," and do nothing, absolutely nothing, about it except from useless bureaucratic agencies which get their supporters jobs and encourage people to turn in their enemies (whether they are using dope or not).

Well, as I see it, we've got two choices: A. We make heroin legal and let the people who want to use it do so without robbing, stealing, and being generally disagreeable to support the habit (very, very few crimes are commited by nodding junkies. They are committed by "sick" ones who can't work up the bread to score). B. We beat the living shit out of every junkie we see, until the whole game gets too unpopular to attract new users.

"A" would no doubt be the easiest. I mean, who would suffer? The crime

rate would go down by a big jump, the generally useless people who become junkies would be out of the way and not bothering anyone or raising politically felt havoc, the scummy types who make their living out of selling smack would be out of business, big crime would lose a fortune, and almost everyone would be happy.

The problem is no politician wants to go on record as being "in favor" of drugs. Regardless of the fact that the program works well in England, it still seems like an extreme (or a soft, depending on your political affiliation) method of cutting crime. Who knows, maybe the pawnshop owners have a powerful lobby, and they are preventing this idea from becoming reality, or maybe the Mafia is. . .

So we have "B". Now here is an active grass-roots political program that all of us who crave action and social change could get invovled with. We would simply band together and check out people who appear to be under the influence: look at his pupils, smell his breath. Is he just tired or drunk? Any tracks? If so, we should descend on him like the sea gulls did on the locusts in Salt Lake.

Stones, clubs, and fists should rain upon the offender until he is beaten senseless and driven back to his scummy hideaway. Train school children to spot doorway nodders and stone them. Give little old ladies clubs.

Maybe this approach is the real answer. As it stands now, there is just too much "understanding" and tolerance floating around. The politician riding in his limo and living upon the hill doesn't get ripped off, so he understands the problem and the "sickness" that causes it.

No, it's you and me, the man on the street, the little old lady with her purse, that suffer the consequences. We must realize that the junkie is not a part of our environment.

For as the system's scientist defines environment, (i.e. that which affects our way of life, but is outside our control) the junkie does not fit. He can be controlled. If the political forces that be will not succumb to the Orwellian notion of a happy and drugged-out lower class, we must change the situation in another way.

Pick up a club.

Acupuncture is coming into vogue as a partial treatment for heroin addiction. The technique consists of sticking an acupuncture needle into the patient's outer ear and wiggling it about with much vigor.

Reportedly this relieves, at least to some extant, the symptoms of a hard withdrawal.

A Los Angeles clinic has modified this procedure by applying a local anesthetic to the ear and then clipping a steel staple at the needle point. The addict is then motivated to wiggle the staple, with the same vigor, three or four times a day. This achieves the same symptomatic relief.

A mass implementing of this idea would achieve many side sociological effects as well: drug addicts would all be effectively "branded", making it easy to publically identify such creatures, job interviewers would have a markedly easier job, and finding people to fill sparse police lineups would be one heck of a lot simpler.

Of course, we could also expect a reverse backlash wherein the magic staple would take on a status symbol quality, people would be selling fake clips under the counter in fine jewelry stores, rock musicians and other heavies would start to wear a clip in each ear, people might well begin wiggling each other's clips in search of wierd sexual thrills, and suburban high schools would no doubt experience a rash of people getting clipped to each other for the big dance.............

The physiological treatment for drug (primarily heroin) addiction takes three major approaches:

Replacement — Use of a synthetic, opiate-like drug which alleviates the necessity of heroin, yet lacks (or some, depending on your viewpoint) of the negative side effects. Methadone is the most effective drug in this category.

Antagonistic — Similar to the use of Anti-use in chronic alcoholic cases; a drug is injected into the subject on a daily (may bet getter) basis. If the subject then uses an opiate based drug, he will experience sort of a medical bad karma. . .usually, this takes the form of vomiting, minor convulsions, and other non-joyful manifestations. The theory being that the user wants to avoid the bad reaction to a healthy enough degree that he will avoid the opiate drug. The trick here, of course, is to get the chronic user to continue to take his daily bread. This is encouraged by threats (the VA is reportedly using a program of this type) of no help, no benefits, or even jail. A longer lasting antagonist, whereby the injection would produce the bad reaction for some time, say weeks, afterwards, would help the weak willed. . .

The third, and probably the avenue that shows the most promise, is the use of a drug which counters the withdrawal symptoms and to some extent, the craving which accompanies a cold turkey approach. The newest and first drug which actually seems to do just this is Darvon N; reportedly a combination of Darvon (a common pain killer) and Aspirin. Darvon N seems to alleviate up to 100% of the withdrawal symptoms and greatly reduces the need for heroin. It is non-habit forming and has few negative side effects.

(continued from p. 81)

dangerous to kick than barbiturates or possibly even Quaalude. A cold turkey withdrawal will clean the body out in about three days.

The kicking is not fun to be sure – cold sweats, pains, tremors, depression, puking, and other exciting things, but the side effects, such as seizures are likely to be small and not deadly.

The main danger is that the addict, feeling so lousy for the next month or so, will shoot up to relieve the problems.

Withdrawal can be eased by methadone, a synthetic narcotic, which arrives from accessible to illegal in various parts of the country. Methadone works as a treatment if people know how to use it, and no one really does.

The megavitamin therapy described in the OD-Wipeout section of this book seems to help ease the withdrawal symptoms and craving more than anything else short of methadone.

LSD

Lysergic acid diethylamine is a semisynthetic hallucinogen made from a chemical synthesized from a rye fungus called Claviceps purpurea. This fungus is a parasitic disease which attacks rye plants. A closely related type of lysergic acid is found in several versions of morning glory seeds, (see legal highs section).

LSD was commercially "invented" in 1938 by two research chemists working for Sandoz labs in Switzerland. One of the chemists accidentally ingested the drug and experienced a "kind of drunken – although not unpleasant state, which was characterized by extreme imagination". This was undoubtedly the first good trip.

Not knowing the dosage he had taken, the chemist tried to repeat the experiment with a dose of 250 micrograms and fell into a severe drunkenlike state in which he began "shouting insanely and babbling." Dr. Hoffman, thus, became the first man to experience both a good and a bad acid trip.

The normal dosage of PURE laboratory LSD is 25 – 30 mics. At about 35 and over, most classic schizophrenialike symptoms begin to appear. When the doses reach the 400 – 500 stage, there is an increase in blood pressure, sweating, a marked increase in pupil size, tremors of the extremities. These dosages reflect the classic definition of strychnine added to LSD, when in actuality, the drug is usually just a massive overdose of LSD.

A half teaspoonful of salt weighs about 2.4 grams. This is equal to 2,400 milligrams and 2,400,000 doses per gram, at 50 cents a dose, *equals about $5,760,000, and you ask why I did it?"*

ED. NOTE: The outcome of this philosophy was quite predictable — he went to prison, but still you've got to respect his honesty.)

The average gram of acid (28.8 grams to the ounce) is usually figured out to make about 4,000 tablets. This means (not counting any loss, which of course, there is a bit) about 250 mics a tab — a hell of a dose if the batch turns out to be nearly pure and the losses are minimized.

Unfortunately, it is very hard to uniformly distribute a dosage as small as this in a quantity of cutting material. The same batch of acid can produce both good and bad trips since a (pure) dosage of 25 — 30 is considered a good dosage. Levels of 70 — 100 mics will go either way, and levels of over 300 micrograms will produce consistently bad trips, many of which will equate strychnine poisoning symptoms.

LSD has a definite tolerance level. This level begins to show up in as soon as four trips. After this point, it takes an ever-increasing (up to a leveling-off point) dose to produce the same reaction. If the chemist or his guinea pig has a high tolerance level because of frequent ingesting, the tabs may get superdoses of acid.

In analyzing HUNDREDS of lab reports from testing centers all over the country, we have found only one or maybe two cases that actually contained strychnine. FOR ALL PRACTICAL PURPOSES, THERE IS NO STRYCHNINE IN LSD IN AMERICA.

LSD presents a problem with respect to setting up doses as the quantities are so minute as to make weighing or dividing highly inaccurate. The first noncommercially produced acid may have well appeared in the form of drops or in sugar cubes. One cube was usually about 45 — 50 mics and normally a good trip. This early acid was quite consistent and often associated with Leary and Owsley, the "fathers" of the acid movement.

As the word got around, sugar cubes became more obvious and tended to decompose too quickly. The sophisticated sellers switched to capping. This was accomplished by figuring out how much inert filler (usually lactose or Similac) would fill the required number of capsules (usually between 2,000 — 4,000) and mixing the gram of acid in the filler. This resulted in a highly uneven spread of the drug throughout the filler and could mean a weak trip one time and a superheavy trip the next. As the rip-off artists began to appear, the capsule began falling into disfavor because of the ease in which any substance could be shoved into a gelatin cap and sold as acid.

Tabbing began to come into use about this stage. The tabbing machine was usually a commercial machine and hard to get hold of. The mixing procedures were better and the doses more consistent. The buyer tended to trust the tablet more as it indicated a higher form of sophistication in the manufacturing process and probably a better grade of LSD. Tabbers began to strive for individuality by "signing" their products with a particular symbol; peace signs, crosses, lines, and variations in shape such as the mini, the barrel, the flat, etc. This began to mark each particular chemist. Each batch would also be colorcoded with an identifiable color. If the batch sold well and got a good reputation, it would be continued. If it produced bummers or got an otherwise undesirable name, it could quickly be discontinued and another color substituted. This would give the chemist a breather to get rid of the bad batch before the word got around on the new color.

The amateurs began finding it harder and harder to sell untabbed products and began to imitate the better operations, usually without a tabbing machine to rely on.

One method was to dissolve the gram of acid in a small quantity of vodka (acid is alcohol soluable) and drop or "splash" the liquid LSD onto already existing tablets. A favorite was the drugstore vitamin C tabs. Often, the drop-ons would be colored to produce some method of authenticity. Probably the most famous example of this was the "purple splash," widely circulated during the late Haight-Ashbury days.

Another reason different manufacturers strived for individuality in packaging was the increase in competition, and some notable examples came up (most of which didn't require a tabbing machine, as the narcs were now keeping close tabs on anyone trying to purchase a tabbing machine for any purpose). Some famous efforts in this direction were/are "clear light" acid dropped on clear gelatin "window panes"; blotter acid (which has reappeared again and again in a variety of colors and sizes), where the liquid acid is dropped on small squares of blotter paper and usually sold by the inch. Occasionally, offbeat examples would show up such as the bubble gum craze in San Francisco, the chocolate acid craze in Colorado, liquid acid in small vials in Florida, etc., but most of these soon became outdated due to the difficulty in storage and other inherent problems. There was one Denver, Colorado, chemist who was known for putting his best batches with chloral hydrate (a tranquilizer) and painting it on ping pong balls with the word "BOO." This "blue boo" was all the rage for the in-freaks, one letter was said to equal about 50 mics.

Probably the most famous, consistently good, form of acid was orange sunshine, which later graduated into orange barrel acid. This was associated with the "Brotherhood," a large, well-stocked smuggling/manufacturing group, of which Leary was a reputed member. The original sunshine was supposedly made by Owsley himself and seemed to follow the Grateful Dead from town to town on their tours. Whenever the Brotherhood was busted, the acid in the area took a drop in quality. Probably no acid has been copied as much as sunshine or orange barrels.

Clear light is probably the only form of LSD which has been present in the same form from the same group of people for several years. Clear light comes packaged in the form of small, clear gelatin squares which contain pure, usually quite high quality LSD. The squares have been packaged in small heat-sealed plastic tubes at one hundred hits per tube, but have recently switched to recappable tubes. It is sold from the chemist in one gram lots, usually going for about $1,300 per gram and comes in handcrafted miniboxes, mainly wooden.

It is made in Northern California, and although the locations have switched several times in the last few years, it is still around the San Francisco Bay area.

It appears to be semisynthetic acid and the quality remains quite constant. This has, in turn, spawned several counterfeiters, some of whom have tried to use the original Clear light format, and some of whom have altered it slightly, as in colored "windowpane" acid. Such as the "notched green triangle" which is circulating at the time of this writing.

The microdot tabs (where the chemical is/was concentrated in one small, colored area on the tab) have pretty much run the gamut of every conceivable color and shape as has the speckled (where a couple of different colors make up the tab in a conglomerate arrangement).

Undoubtedly, the most famous acid, for the real freak, has to be the clear caps signed with a Z or even an owl . . . but they, too, have retired to the elephant's graveyard. (Stories still circulate in San Francisco about the times Owsley used to come into the city to go to his bank – here would be this freaky person in bare feet pulling 20 dollar bills from every orifice in his wardrobe and laying them on the counter. Inevitably, he would have his main collection in his motorcycle helmet).

Throughout the years, acid has been mixed and marketed with a variety of other drugs. Speed/acid combinations were the rage for a short while, although now acid is being mixed with PCP with a bit more frequency than with speed. Usually though, LSD being sold for

LSD is just that, in quantities ranging from 20 to 500 mics. About 50 per cent of street acid seems to be fairly impure, maybe enough to cause a fair percentage of bummers.

Occasionally, capsules can indicate a second operation where the tab is crushed and adulterated with a cut and sold in weaker doses. This is particularly true when a strong batch of acid hits the streets.

LSD use is falling off, per se. However, total LSD sales, due to the fact that LSD and LSD/PCP combinations are being increasingly sold as other drugs, are actually on the rise. It is estimated that acid has leveled off to about ten million doses per year.

LSD does not cause significant chromosome damage. It does cause breakage in the chromosomes, but at not much greater rate than aspirin, caffeine, color TV, etc. do.

Acid should NEVER be taken by people who are manic depressives, or anyone in a down state of mind, as it has the effect of amplifying emotions many times. LSD tends to strip away the ego layer of the human personality. This can be disastrous to someone who is used to seeing himself through conditioning layers and does not accept the real "himself." People HAVE landed in mental institutions from one use of fairly mild LSD.

LSD is sometimes cut with garbage, near-psychedelics, left over from the manufacturing process. This produces a more physical reaction, usually in the form of a speedy trip, but not usually too strong.

LSD is usually made by mixing lysergic acid with diethylamide, freezing the mixture, and then extracting by fractional distillation with chloroform, benezine, or a vacuum pump. For this reason, it is almost impossible to get lysergic acid (the FDA made it illegal to own without an FDA number and then made it impossible to get for just about any reason) and smuggled lysergic acid, often from Italy, occasionally from Canada, runs $1,000 – $5,000 a liter. The narcs also tend to watch people who attempt to buy vacuum pumps.

The accepted theory of LSD action is that it acts to block the catecholamines or replaces them in the brain. This breaks down the normal routes of communication from parts of the body to the brain, so that the brain is deluged with unusual sensory stimuli in many startling ways. It also seems to affect the amine levels as with MOA inhibitors and may cause some long-term bodily changes until the levels return to normal.

At one time this was thought to cause "flashbacks," where the brain was triggered to produce the trip sensations without any drug, but it is now believed that "flashbacks" occur very infrequently, and may happen only to schizophrenia-prone persons. Since schizophrenia closely resembles low key acid trips, reemerging schizophrenia may be incorrectly classified as flashbacks.

Only a small percentage of LSD actually enters the brain (about .01 per cent), and this is usually out of the brain in 20 minutes. Therefore, it stands to reason, that its action on nerve cells must be partly or completely indirect. The rest of the dose goes into the kidneys, skin, liver, heart, muscles, etc., and can be detected by an EEG as long as six days after use. The detectable level (as in BUST) leaves the bloodstream in about two hours from the time of use.

LSD usually takes effect ½ to 1½ hours after ingestion and may last from 6 to 14 hours. It has been also found to increase the amount of serotonin in brain cells. Following the trip, there is a crash or depression period, but not as bad as with speed. LSD is not an aphrodisiac, but does lower one's inhibitions.

There is no physical dependence or withdrawal symptoms. However, a tolerance does appear and it is an effective cross-tolerance to mescaline and psilocybin, but not speed. (This means it will take a larger dose of either of the three drugs, should a tolerance level be built up for one of them).

Some users dig the trip to the effect that an effective psychological dependence is built up. Some however, find the experience so intense that they have no desire to repeat it frequently.

The usual trip is hard to put into words, but common reactions include: intensified colors and sounds, a crossing of the sense known as "synthesia," in which one may see tastes or hear colors, etc. There is a loss of the time sense and sound. The relationship between current stimuli and past experience is lost. Feelings and emotions are heightened and behavior altered. The ego is stripped away and the person can find himself fused with his surroundings or with other people. There is a general feeling of increased creativity, but this is not proven to be true.

It is an hallucinogenic drug, but NOT ALL users will hallucinate. These hallucinations can take the form of vivid colors, swirling images, meeting of lines, shapes distorted, objects falling apart, and so on.

Because of the minimal dose required, the drug is considered one of the most potent known to man.

Negative reactions usually happen in three types of users:

1. Unstable persons harboring a latent psychosis.

2. People who have been turned on without their knowledge.

3. People who take the drug in a hostile or unnatural environment.

For more particulars on this, see the bummers' section.

In one of the rare instances of a major drug company feeling any pangs of conscience, Sandoz Manufacturing Company, the only legit supplier of LSD in the States, quit making the drug due to adverse publicity and the fact that their drug was falling into the wrong hands.

GROWING LSD

Due to the difficulty in securing lysergic acid, much of the underground LSD is made from this "semiorganic" process. The basic culture here is Claviceps purpurea. This is purchased from biological supply houses or secured directly from the field where it occurs naturally on rye grass. The ergot is a disease which attacks rye grass and appears as a blackish growth on the tops of the rye grasses where the seeds are. They are about the same shape as the seeds themselves. From the tips of there ergot "heads" sprouts the Claviceps purpurea fungi. When viewed under a strong microscope, they have long stems and bulbous heads.

When the field method is used, the chemist must remove this fungi from the heads of the ergot and maintain it under sterile conditions. This stuff is potentially dangerous and should not be handled by those who do not know how to deal with poisonous compounds such as ergots.

The chemist usually employs a commercial agar solution or makes one from: sucrose — 100 grams, chick pea meal — 50 grams, calcium nitrate — 1 gram, potassium chloride — 125 grams, ferrous sulphate heptahydrate — 8.35 milligrams, zinc sulphate heptahydrate — 3.5 milligrams. This mixture is dissolved in distilled water to totally equal one quart and adjusted to a pH of 4 with an ammonia solution and citric acid. It must be autoclaved to achieve sterilization.

The Claviceps purpurea is innoculated into this medium under sterile conditions and allowed to incubate for two weeks. During this time the pH of 4 must be maintained.

Several one gallon jugs are often used to grow the mixture by preparing them as follows: A two-holed stopper is placed in the jug's neck, and a piece of 6-inch glass tubing is placed in one of the holes, with about two inches protruding above the surface. A piece of rubber tubing is attached to the glass tube.

Fill a small (500) milliliter Erlenmeyer flask with a dilute solution of sodium hypochlorite and extend a glass tube from the rubber tube so the end is immersed in the hypochlorite. Fit a long glass tube in the other stopper hole. It must reach near the bottom of the jug and have about two inches showing above the stopper. Attach a rubber tube to the glass tube as short or as long as desired and fit a short glass tube to the end of the rubber tube. Fill a large glass tube (1 inch by 6 inches) with sterile cotton and fit 1-hole stoppers in the ends. Fit another small glass tube in the other stopper. A rubber tube is connected to this and attached to a small air pump obtained from a tropical fish supply store. One now has a setup for pumping air from the pump, through the cotton filter, down the long glass tube in the jug, through the solution to the air space in the top of the jugs, through the short glass tube, down to the bottom of the Erlenmeyer flask, and up through the sodium hypocholorite solution into the atmosphere. With this aeration equipment one can assure a supply of clean air to the Claviceps purpurea fungus while maintaining a sterile atmosphere inside the solution.

Take the whole mess apart and sterilize in the autoclave.

Fill the jugs about ¾ full of the mixture and autoclave.

Blend the culture you have all together to use for incubation purposes. Everything must be sterile.

Assemble everything and start the pumps. A slow bubbling is enough to provide the culture with oxygen.

Everything must remain in a dark room at room temperature for about ten days.

After this growth period, the culture is adjusted to 1 per cent ethanol using 95 per cent ethanol under sterile conditions.

Now growth is resumed for two weeks.

After this total 24-day period, the culture is made slightly acidic with tartaric acid and mixed thoroughly in a blender for ½ hour.

Then it is adjusted to pH 9 with ammonium hydroxide and extracted with benzene.

Now it is again extracted with alcoholic tartaric acid and evaporated in a vacuum to dryness. This dry material is the salt of the ergot alkaloids and is stored in this form by most underground chemists.

CONVERSION OF AMIDES

The amides can be recovered for conversion to LSD by making it basic with ammonia (pH of 9) and extracted with chloroform and evaporated in a vacuum.

Often an unexperienced chemist will stop here. The amide can be packaged and sold, although the dose is a bit unstable, normally about one milligram of amide will produce the reaction of 100 micrograms of LSD.

The extraction of LSD from the amide is a potentially dangerous process *with poisonous fumes and possibly explosive mixtures of vapors and air. The publishers of this book do NOT advise you to attempt any of the processes given here, as they are given for information ONLY. However, we especially urge you not to attempt the reduction to LSD.*

REDUCTION TO LSD

Dissolve ten grams of the amide in 200 milliliters of methanolic potassium hydroxide solution.

Remove the methanol by vacuum as soon as the above step is completed.

Dissolve the residue into 200 milliliters of an 8 per cent solution of potassium hydroxide in water. Heat this mixture in a steam bath for one hour.

Pass a stream of nitrogen gas through the flask in the heating process.

Neutralize the mixture with tartaric acid and run it through filter paper.

Extract the mixture with ether in a separatory funnel saving the water layer and throwing away the ether layer.

Filter the solution through filter paper and evaporate.

Dry crystals of LSD will remain.

MARIJUANA

Marijuana is a deciduous plant which grows from seeds. The fibrous section of the plant was (has been replaced by synthetics) used to make rope. The flowering tops, leaves, seeds, and resin of the plant is used by jazz musicians, freaks, and other social outcasts to get HIGH.

Normally, the vegetable parts of the plant are smoked to produce this "high," but they can also be eaten. The active ingredient in marijuana resin is THC (tetrahydrocannabinol). Marijuana contains from 1 - 4 per cent THC (4 per cent must be considered GOOD dope).

Marijuana grows wild in many parts of the world, and is cultivated in Mexico, Vietnam, Africa, Nepal, India, South America, etc., etc. The marijuana sold in the United States comes primarily from, yes, the United States.

It is estimated that at least 50 per cent of the grass on the streets in America is homegrown. The next largest bunch comes across the borders from Mexico, with smaller amounts filtering in from Panama, occasionally South America, and occasionally, Africa.

(continued on p. 100)

CHEMISTRY

This book is NOT designed to make you a chemist (or if you are a chemist, it is not designed to make you an underground chemist), there are MUCH more detailed books on the subject available to the buyer. With the exception of the few THC extraction formulas and organic drug syntheses presented here, no one could possibly make drugs from our simple text, right?

At any rate, as previously stated, WE DO NOT suggest that you attempt any of these processes, and they are, by and large, illegal, dangerous, and difficult.

HOWEVER, if you do feel this incredible urge to do so, in spite of our warnings, you should be aware of a couple of facts:

Narcs and chemical companies cooperate with the diligence of lovers. If you attempt to order such drugs as P_2P *(phenyl-2-proponone), Indole, lithium aluminum hydrite, olivetol, and ergotamine, you can just about be sure that you have called the attention of the DEA to be thrown in your humble direction.*

At some companies, the ordering of a mere vacuum pump (especially, if you do not look like a normal, everyday, straight chemist and/or have a good cover story) will lead to trouble.

NEVER, NEVER, NEVER give your real name, address, etc. Expect them to attempt to take your picture (under cover, of course) and check for people following you to your car to get license numbers and possibly following you out of the lab parking lot.

Labs will often fill a small portion of your order, just enough for one batch of whatever, and let the DEA bust you, as not to give the name of the profession which makes napalm, nerve gas, mace and other good things, a bad name.

There are a couple of chemical hints which can be useful in psychedelic manufacture: DRYING can be accomplished with an anhydrous salt, such as $MgSO_4$ *and filtering out the salt. Solids or residues can be dried in room temperature or in a low heat oven.*

Petroleum ether is NOT regular ether and the two CANNOT be substituted.

Vacuum extraction normally requires an expensive and suspicious vacuum pump, but for most drug chemistry, a simple water-source vacuum will suffice.

Stirring can be done by hand in an emergency, but a magentic stirrer is almost a necessity.

Heating: NEVER heat over an open flame or have any open flame in the same room (pilot lights, water heaters, people smoking, etc.). Heating plates can be used, but an electric flask heating mantle is by far the best.

If you do not have a lab ventilating hood, use a fan with an open window.

ALWAYS use gloves, tongs, and a face shield of unbreakable plastic.

CAN YOU REALLY BUY ANYTHING IN MEXICAN JAILS?

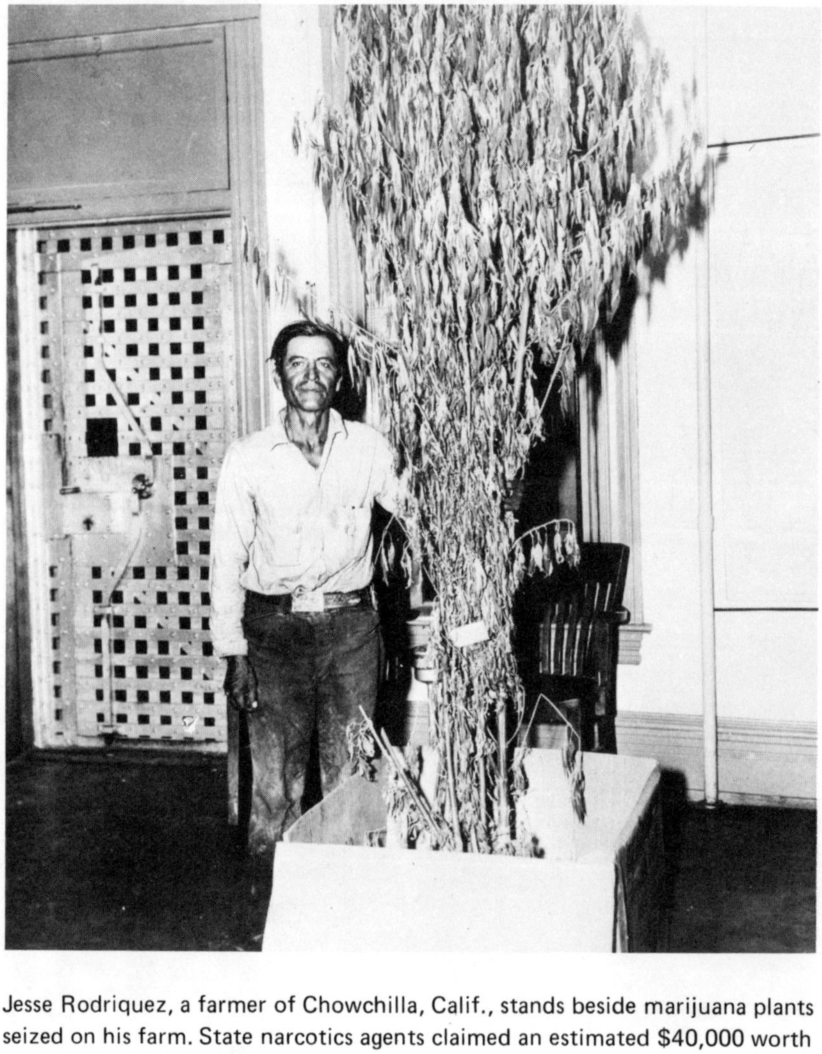

Jesse Rodriquez, a farmer of Chowchilla, Calif., stands beside marijuana plants seized on his farm. State narcotics agents claimed an estimated $40,000 worth of marijuana was found growing between ears of corn.

World Wide Photos

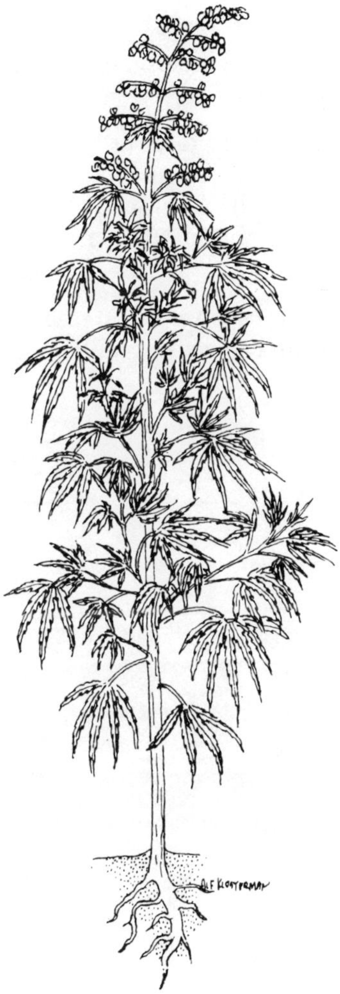

God grows his own. The magic weed in all its glory . . . .

(continued from p. 95)

Hashish is the pure resin of the marijuana plant, which is scraped from the flowering tops of the plant and lumped together. Ganja is the ground-up tops of the finest plants. (It is also the name given to any sort of marijuana in Jamaica.)

Marijuana will deteriorate in about two years if exposed to light, air or heat. It should always be stored in cool places.

Grass prices in the United States are a direct reflection of the laws of supply and demand (and you thought that high school economics would never be useful). A series of large border busts, a short growing season, a bad crop, any number of things can drive the price of marijuana up.

Demand still seems to be on the increase in the U.S., so prices seldom fall below last year's level.

MARYGIN:

Marygin is an anagram of the words marijuana and gin, as in Eli Whitney. It is a plastic tumbler which acts much like a commercial cotton gin.

One takes about one ounce of an herb and breaks it up. This is then placed in the Marygin and the protruding knob is rotated. This action turns the internal wheel, which separates the grass from the debris (seeds, stems).

It does not pulverize the grass as screens have a habit of doing and is easily washable.

Marygin is available from:

P.O. Box 5827
Tucson, Arizona 85703
$5.00

Each year a small seasonal drought occurs, as last year's supply runs low, and next year's crop is not up yet. Prices usually rise about 20 – 75 per cent during this time and then fall back to "normal."

Unquestionably, a large shortage of grass causes a percentage of smokers to turn to harder drugs instead. For this reason, no grass control program can ever be beneficial or "successful."

GROW IT!

There is one surefire way of avoiding high prices and the grass DT's: Grow your own. This is not as difficult as some "authorities" on the subject would make you believe. Marijuana is a weed, and a fairly vivacious one at that, and it will grow almost in spite of you.

OUTDOORS

Contrary to popular belief, grass grows well in many places on the North American continent. It will flourish even if the temperature does not rise above 75 degrees.

The plants do need a minimum of eight hours of sunlight per day and should be planted in late April/early May, BUT DEFINITELY, after the last frost of the year.

Growing an outdoor, or "au naturel", crop has been the favored method over the years, because grass seems to grow better without as much attention, when in its natural habitat.

Of course, an outdoors setting requires special precautions not encountered with an indoors crop; you must be able to avoid detection, both from law enforcement freaks and common freaks, both of whom will take your weed and probably use it. Of course, one will also arrest you. You must also have access to the area to prepare the soil and harvest the crop.

There are two schools of thought about starting the seeds. One says you should start the seedlings for about ten days in an indoor starter box (see the indoor section) and then transplant. The other theory is that you should just start them in the correct location. Fewer plants will come up with this method, but there is no shock of transplant to kill some of the seedlings halfway through.

The soil should be preprepared for the little devils by turning it over a couple of times and adding about one cup of hydrated lime per square yard of soil and a little bit (not too much, now) of good water soluble nitrogen fertilizer. The soil should now be watered several times and left to sit about one week.

The plants should be planted at least three feet apart, getting too greedy and stacking them too close will result in stunted plants.

The plants like some water during their growing season, BUT not too much. This is especially true around the roots, as too much water will rot the root system.

Grass grows well with corn or hops, and these plants will help provide some camouflage. It does not grow well with rye, spinach, or pepperweed.

It is probably a good idea to plant in many small, broken patches, as people tend to notice patterns.

GENERAL GROWING INFO

Both the male and female plant produce THC resin, although the male is not as strong as the female. In a good crop, the male will still be plenty smokable and should not be thrown away under any circumstances.

Marijuana can reach a height of twenty feet (or would you rather wish on a star) and obtain a diameter of 4½ inches. If normal, it has a sex ratio of about 1:1, but this can be altered in several ways.

The male plant dies in the 12th week of growing, the female will live another 3 – 5 weeks to produce her younguns. Females can weigh twice as much as males when they are mature.

Marijuana soil should compact when you squeeze it, but should also break apart with a small pressure and absorb water well. A nice test for either indoor or outdoor growing is to add a bunch of worms to the soil, if they live and hang around, it is good soil, but if they don't, well, change it. Worms also help keep the soil loose enough for the plants to grow well.

SEEDS

To get good grass, you should start with the right seeds. A nice starting point is to save the seeds from the best bunch you have consumed. The seeds should be virile, that is, they should not be grey and shriveled up, but green, meaty, and healthy appearing. A nice test is to drop the seeds on a hot frying pan. If they "CRACK," they are probably good for planting purposes.

The seeds should be soaked in distilled water overnight before planting. BE SURE to plant in the ground with the pointy end UP. Plant about ½" deep.

Healthy seeds will sprout in about five days.

SPROUTING

The best all around sprouting method is probably to make a sprouting box (as sold in nurseries) with a slated bottom or use paper cups with holes punched in the bottoms. The sprouting soil should be a mixture of humus, soil, and fine sand with a bit of organic fertilizer and water mixed in about one week before planting.

When ready to transplant, you must be sure and leave a ball of soil around the roots of each plant. This whole ball is dropped into a baseball-sized hole in the permanent soil.

If you are growing/transplanting indoors, you should use a green safe light (purchased at nurseries) during the transplanting operation. If you are transplanting outdoors, you should time it about two hours before sunset to avoid damage to the plant. Always wear cotton gloves when handling the young plants.

After the plants are set in the hole, you should water them. It is also a good idea to use a commercial transplant chemical (also purchased at nurseries) to help them overcome the shock.

INDOOR GROWING

Indoor growing has many advantages, besides the apparent fact that it is much harder to have your crop "found," you can control the ambient conditions just exactly as you want them and get a guaranteed "good" plant.

Plants grown indoors will not appear the same as their outdoor cousins. They will be scrawnier appearing with weak stems and may even require you to tie them to a growing post to remain upright, BUT THEY WILL HAVE AS MUCH OR MORE RESIN!

If growing in a room, you should put tar paper on the floors and then buy sterilized bags of soil from a nursery. You will need about one cubic foot of soil for each plant.

The plants will need about 150 ml. of water per plant/per week. They will also need fresh air, so the room must be ventilated. (However, the fresh air should contain NO TOBACCO smoke.)

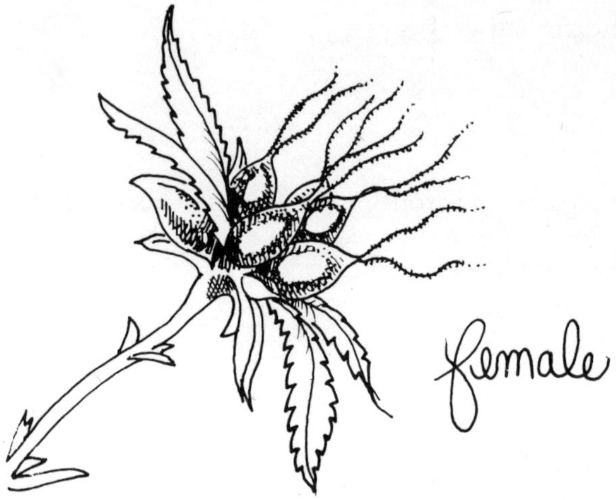

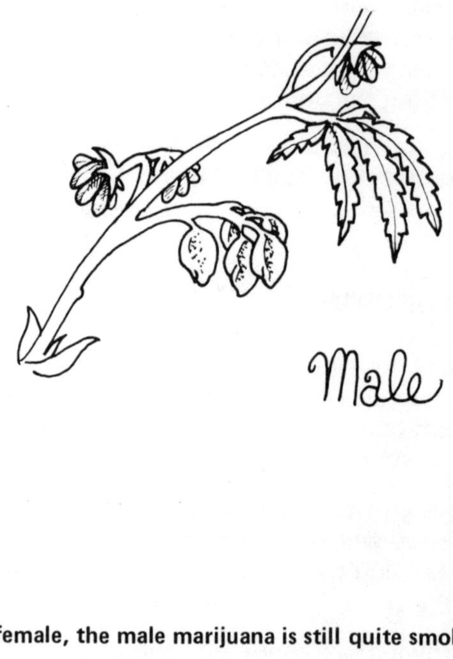

While not as potent as the female, the male marijuana is still quite smokable...

At least eight hours of light a day must be provided. As you increase the light, the plants grow faster and show more females/less males. Sixteen hours of light per day seems to be the best combination, beyond this makes little or no appreciable difference in the plant quality. Another idea is to interrupt the night cycle with about one hour of light. This gives you more females.

The walls of your growing room should be painted white or covered with aluminum foil to reflect the light.

The lights themselves can be either bulbs or fluorescent. Figure about 75 watts per plant or one plant per two feet of flourescent tube. The fluorescents are the best, but do not use "cool white" types. The light sources should be an average of twenty inches from the plant and NEVER closer than 14 inches. They may be mounted on a rack and moved every few days as the plants grow.

The very best light sources are those made by Sylvania and others especially for growing plants (such as the "gro lux" types).

HARVESTING AND DRYING

The male plants will be taller and have about five green or yellow sepals, which will split open to fertilize the female plant with pollen.

The female plant is shorter and has a small pistillate flower, which really doesn't look like a flower at all but rather a small bunch of leaves in a cluster.

If you don't want any seeds, just good dope, you should pick the males before they shed their pollen as the female will use some of her resin to make the seeds.

After another three to five weeks, after the males are gone, the females will begin to wither and die (from loneliness?), this is the time to pick.

In some nefarious Middle Eastern countries, farmers reportedly put their beehives next to fields of marijuana. The little devils collect the grass pollen for their honey, which is supposed to contain a fair dosage of THC.

The honey is then enjoyed by conventional methods or made into ambrosia.

If you want seeds — let the male shed his pollen and then pick him. Let the female go about another month and pick her.

To cure the plants, they must be dried. On large crops, this is

(continued on p. 109)

YES, VIRGINIA, YOU CAN MAKE BEER FROM THE HOPS GRASS CONVERSION, AND SOME OF THE GOOD STUFF IS BROUGHT ALONG FOR THE RIDE...

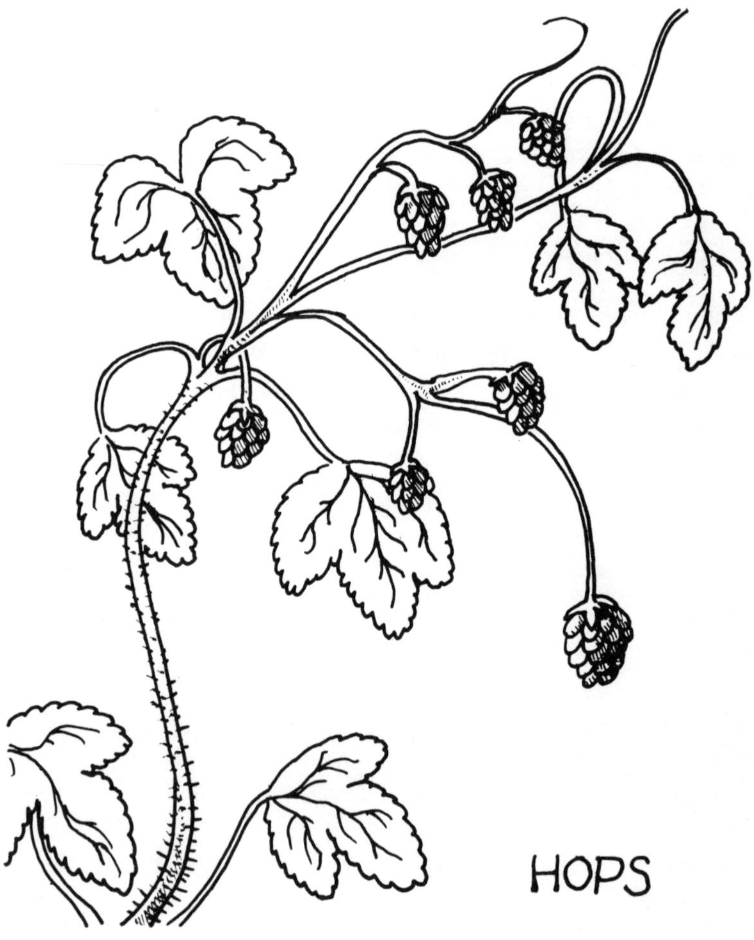

HOPS

PLANT PROBLEM CHART

Always check the overall environmental conditions prior to passing judgment – soil around 7 pH or slightly less – plenty of water, light, fresh air, loose soil, no water standing in pools.

SYMPTOM	PROBABLY PROBLEM/CURE
Larger leaves turning yellow – smaller leaves still green.	Nitrogen deficiency – add nitrate of soda or organic fertilizer.
Older leaves will curl at edges, turn dark, possibly with a purple cast.	Phosphorus deficiency – add commercial phosphate.
Mature leaves develop a yellowish cast to least veinal areas.	Magnesium deficiency – add commercial fertilizer with a magnesium content.
Mature leaves turn yellow and then become spotted with edge areas turning dark grey.	Potassium deficiency – add muriate of potash.
Cracked stems, no healthy support tissue.	Boron deficiency – add any plant food containing boron.
Small wrinkled leaves with yellowish vein systems.	Zinc deficiency – add commercial plant food containing zinc.
Young leaves become deformed, possibly yellowing.	Molybednum deficinecy – use any plant food containing a bit of molybdenum.

In some nefarious Middle Eastern countries, farmers reportedly put their beehives next to fields of marijuana. The little devils collect the grass pollen for their honey, which is supposed to contain a fair dosage of THC.

The honey is then enjoyed by conventional methods or made into ambrosia.

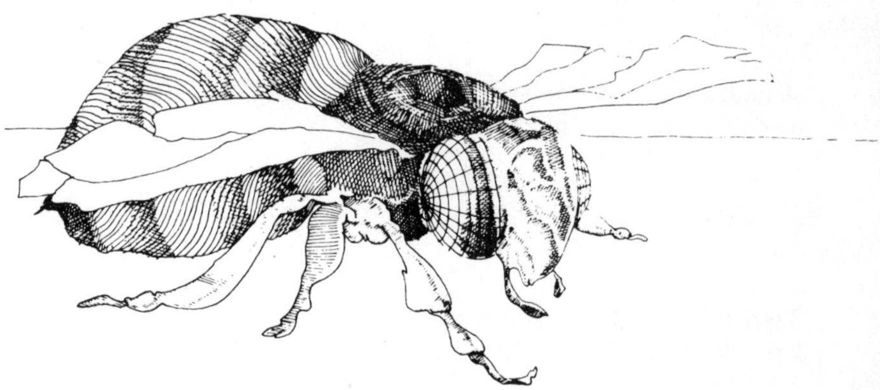

(continued from p. 105)
accomplished by constructing a drying box or drying room.

You must have a heat source (such as an electric heater) which will make the box/room each 130 degrees. The box/room must be ventilated to carry off the water-vapor-laden air and replace it with fresh.

A good box can be constructed from an orange crate with fiberglass insulated walls, vents in the tops, and screen shelves to hold the leaves. There must be a baffle between the leaves and the heat source.

A quick cure for smaller amounts is to: cut the plant at the soil level and wrap it in a cloth so as not to lose any leaves. Take out any seeds by hand and store. Place all the leaves on a cookie sheet or aluminum foil and put them in the middle shelf of the oven, which is set on "broil." In a few seconds, the leaves will smoke and curl up, stir them around and give another ten seconds before you take them out.

TO INCREASE THE GOOD STUFF

There are several tricks to increase the number of females, or the THC content of plants:

You can make the plants mature in 36 days if you are in a hurry, by cutting back on the light to about 14 hours, but the plants will not be as big. You should gradually shorten the light cycle until you reach fourteen hours.

You can stop any watering as the plants begin to make the resin rise to the flowers. This will increase the resin a bit.

You can use a sunlamp on the plants as they begin to develop flower stalks.

You can snip off the flower, right at the spot where it joins the plant, and a new flower will form in a couple of weeks. This can be repeated two or three times to get several times more flowers than usual.

If the plants are sprayed with Ethrel early in their growth stage, they will produce almost all female plants. This usually speeds up the flowering also, it may happen in as little as two weeks.

You can employ a potent growth changer called colchicine. This is a bit hard to get and expensive. (Should be ordered through a lab of some sort and costs about $35 a gram.)

GRASS

Edmund Scientific Company
555 Edscorp Building
Barrington, New Jersey 08007
Free Catalog

is a wonder of good things for the potential grass grower. They have an electric thermostat greenhouse for starting plants for a mere $14.95.

Soil test kits for PH – $2.40

Al tests – $9.95

Soil thermometer – $2.75

Lights which approximate the true color balance of the sun and are probably the most beneficial types available: 40 watt, 48 inch – 4 for $15.75.

Indoor sun bulb, 75 or 150 watt – $5.75.

And, they have a natural growth regulator for plants (Gibberellin) which can change height, speed growth, and maturity, promote blossoming, etc. Each plant reacts differently to treatment with Gibberellin. . .there's no fun like experimenting – $2.00.

To use the colchicine, you should prepare your presoaking solution of distilled water with about 0.10 per cent colchicine. This will cause many of the seeds to die and not germinate, but the ones that do come up will be polyploid plants. This is the accepted difference between such strains as "gold" and normal grass, and yours will DEFINITELY be superweed.

The problem here is that colchicine is a poison in large quantities and may be poisonous in the first generation of plants. Bill Drake, author of CONNOISSEUR'S HANDBOOK OF MARIJUANA runs a very complete colchicine treatment down and warns against smoking the first generation plants (all succeeding generations will also be polyploid) because of this poisonous quality.

However, the Medical Index shows colchicine being given in very small quantities to people for treatment of various ailments. Although these quantities are small, they would appear to be larger than any you could receive from smoking a seed-treated plant.

It would be a good idea to buy a copy of CONNOISSEUR'S, if you are planning to attempt this, and read Mr. Drake's complete instructions.

Another still-experimental process to increase the resin is to pinch off the leaf tips as soon as they appear from the time the plant is in the seedling stage on through its entire life-span. This produces a distorted, wrecked-looking plant which would be very difficult to recognize as marijuana. Of course, there is less substance to this plant, but such wrecked creatures have been known to produce so much resin that it crystallizes as strong hash all over the surface of the plant – might be wise to try it on a plant or two and see what happens.

GRASS RECIPES

On a happy-hippy camping trip, you can roast those whole stocks of grass left over from your last crop over an open fire, much as one might do with marshmallows. Do NOT burn the leaves too much. When they appear toasty brown, dip in honey and eat away, right off Mother Nature, so to speak.

BUTTER: Another good way to use the bad parts of the plant (i.e. stalks, seeds, stems) is to extract the isomers of THC into plain ordinary butter, which can then be used in any number of common recipes to give them an uncommon flair.

First take a pot of water and add about ¾ pound of butter and about 2-3 ounces of weed waste (although good weed will also work).

Place the mixture over a low flame and let simmer for the better part of a day. Strain the mixture back and forth into another pot several times and then flush with hot water in the clean pan. Now, place the hot water/butter mixture into the fridge and skim the butter off as it solidifies and rises to the surface. Throw away the weed and the water.

For a cleaner result, the butter can be reheated and restrained.

BHANG: This is an Indian drink usually concocted from the less potent leaves of the bush. One takes about one joint per person of weed and pulverizes it with a rolling pin, blender, etc. into a fine powder. Add a bit of hot water and stir into a paste. Knead the paste for a minute or so and then add more hot water and strain the liquid into some milk. Redo this straining-through-the-grass process several times.

Now add spices to the milk including: cloves, a bit of sugar, ginger, nutmeg, mace, and allspice. A nice euphoric high results from the consumption of this brew.

Grass can be added to any number of good teas and mixed with hot water. Add enough sugar to counter the taste of the grass.

FRITTERS: A good way to use all those ol' seeds from your cleaned lids:

Toast about 1/3 cup of seeds in a lightly oiled frying pan. Shake often as you would with popcorn

Add the toasted seeds to a packaged pancake mix and stir in about a cup of your favorite fruit (canned peaches, apricots, or fresh blueberries, etc.), then fry over a medium heat until done. A good thing for breakfast or late night snacks.

SEED BALLS: Take about a fourth of a lid of grass, including seeds, and roast in the oven until brown. Mash finely with a Vegematic, rolling pin, or some such implement of destruction.

Mix the grass with a few ground almonds, 3 ounces of ground roasted sesame seeds, about ¼ cup of honey, and ¼ teaspoon each of your favorite spices (cinnamon, nutmeg, allspice, ginger are good). Add a bit of water.

Stir all ingredients in a pan until hot. Add one tablespoon of butter and a dash of salt. Mix. Let cool and roll into candy balls about the size of a ping pong ball and roll in toasted sesame seeds until covered. Potent and good.

FUDGE: Ho boy. Light roast ¼ lid in an oven until just browning. Seeds are not too hot in this one.

Mix together with any fudge recipe.

And add some candied fruit sparingly, such as oranges, cherries, etc. to help conceal the taste of the grass.

BROWNIES: An old standby. If made correctly, it is very difficult to distinguish the taste of the grass, but this is a potent mixture.

Chop ½ lid of grass to a fine powder (a Vegematic, rolling pin, or for good results, use a blender), leave out the seeds, especially if you are trying to disguise the taste of the grass.

Mix in a pan (preferably a double pan where the small one sits in a larger one full of boiling water), 2 ounces unsweetened chocolate, 1/3 cup of butter, and the weed. Now beat in one cup of sugar and two whole eggs.

Stir in ¾ cup of fine flour, ½ teaspoon of baking powder, and ¾ teaspoon of salt. A half cup of chopped almonds or walnuts goes well at this point.

Bake at 350 degrees for ½ hour in a greased baking pan.

When cool, you can spread with icing and cut into itty-bitty squares.

A System for Reputedly Improving the Potency and Giving an Aphrodisiac Quality to Grass:

Take a few oranges and store them in a warm, dark, moist place for a couple of weeks, until a powdery blue mold covers the surface of the oranges.

Clean five ounces of grass.

Take any stems, seeds, etc. you have lying around from various endeavors, as well as those from your cleaned five ounces and put them in a large pot and cover the mess with rubbing alcohol.

Cover the pot and heat on an ELECTRIC hotplate until the sauce begins to thicken (about 2-3 hours on medium heat). NEVER use any kind of open burner or flame to heat alcohol, or you may get an unpleasant surprise.

Drain the alcohol into a container, take the soggy stems and such and repeat the procedure with water instead of alcohol. The thickening should take about one hour. An open burner can be used with the water mixture.

Mix the two separate solutions in one container and put back on the hot plate to boil. Lower the temperature as the mixture gets even thicker.

When the consistency of heavy maple syrup is reached, take off the heat and allow to cool. It will appear to unthicken a bit as it cools off. If it is too watery, resume boiling for a while.

Place the cleaned grass (which can be ground almost to powder) into the mixture and stir well until the mixture is like thick mud.

Now, mix in about 1½ teaspoons of the mold. Once again, stir the mixture until all is thoroughly mixed. This stirring will actually resemble kneading clay if the consistency is correct. Don't be afraid to use your hands.

Put the mixture into a plastic bag, roll the bag shut, and seal. Store in a dark place.

In about two weeks, the grass should have developed an ammonia-like smell. At this point, you should spread the mixture in a baking pan and dry in an oven of about 250 degrees. The oven can be turned off periodically and left hot to further dry the mixture.

Will make a powder which is best consumed in a chillum or pipe.

BAD WEED/GOOD WEED

Can you turn bad weed into good weed? Surprisingly enough, the answer to this oft-asked inquiry is, yes!

Like most other things in life, the amount of good you are going to do relates directly to how much effort you are going to put into it. There are no instant, supermarket products which you can spray on Kansas catnip and have wonderweed, but there are a number of simplified, inexpensive processes (Gee, Mr. Wizard!) which will enhance mediocre grass somewhat, and there are a couple of fairly involved processes which will do up even almost-parsley weed into something worth writing home about.

EASIES:

1. Place the dope in a container which allows air to enter in a restricted fashion (such as a can with nail holes punched in its lid) and add a bunch of dry ice, and then place the whole shebang in the freezer for a few days.

This process will add a certain amount of potency to the product, however, this only works with dry ice, if you use normal, everyday freezer ice, you will end up with a soggy mess. . .

2. Take a quantity of grass and dampen it, place it in a Baggie or another socially acceptable container, and store it in a dark, dampish place for a couple of weeks (burying it also seems to work). The grass will develop a mold which tastes a bit harsh, and burns a tiny bit funny, but does increase the potency.

3. Expose the grass to the high intensity light of a sunlamp for a full day or so. Personally, I don't feel that this is worth the effort, but if you just spent $400 of your friend's money for this brick of super-Colombian, right-from-the-President's-personal-stash, and it turns out to be Missouri weed, and you're packing your bags to leave town before the people arrive for their shares, well, you might at least try it. Can't hurt.

4. Take the undesirable portions of your stash (stems, seeds, weak weed, worms, etc.) and place them in a covered pot, with enough rubbing alcohol to cover everything.

Now CAREFULLY boil the mixture on an ELECTRIC stove or lab burner. DO NOT USE GAS — the alcohol is too flammable. After 45 minutes of heat, remove the pot and strain the solids out, SAVING THE ALCOHOL.

Now, repeat the process with the same residuals, but fresh alcohol. When the second boil is over, remove the solids again, combine the two quantities of alcohol and reboil until you have a syrupy mixture.

Now, this syrupy mixture will contain much of the THC formerly hidden in the stems and such. One simply takes this syrup and thoroughly combines it with the grass that one wishes to improve upon.

For more complicated procedures, see the hash/grass oil section. . .

MDA

There are two basic street types of MDA. One is MMDA, a derivative of the common nutmeg, and a speed-based hallucinogen, known as MDA. The latter was discovered in 1933, and seems to be used, as are many other heavy drugs, by the government to "tranquilize the enemy into submission."

Street MDA is very rare. This leaves the door open to LSD/PCP combinations or PCP/speed, etc., as few people could readily identify real MDA.

Generally, MDA is a bit safer drug than MMDA. If either is manufactured correctly, the chances of a bummer are slight. MDA has some hallucinogenic properties, if a large enough dose is taken. MMDA seems to be almost always hallucinogenic, no matter what the dose is.

MMDA is the active constituent of nutmeg. Myristica oil seems to contain about 4 per cent MMDA, which is removed by simple steam distillation. MMDA is about three to four times as potent as mescaline.

Street MDA or MMDA is probably not either drug. Real MDA can be a smooth, rather enjoyable trip, but to find it in the pure state on the street is next to impossible.

MESCALINE

Peyote is a small, buttonlike cactus which occurs naturally in the southwestern part of the United States and far into Mexico. The cactus contains eleven alkaloids, the main one being 3,4,5-trimethoxyphenlethyamine, or as it is commonly referred to – Mescaline.

The buttons are consumed by Indians in various religious rites (which, when you stop to think about it, sounds like a heck of a lot more fun and probably more religious than Sunday school). The Indians normally chew about three to six buttons per experience. One can only surmise that the difference in dose must depend on how sinful a week the Indian had.

The mescaline can be extracted from the peyote, buttons can be eaten by themselves (tastes vaguely like what you would have to imagine dog shit tastes like) or ground up and capped in gelatin capsules to slide by the taste buds. Mescaline can also be synthetically manufactured (usually as mescaline sulfate), but it is considerably more expensive to make than acid and not often done.

Peyote, and to a lesser extent, organic (and to an even lesser extend, synthetic) mescaline, has a tendency to cause a heavy case of nausea in the user just before the trip takes hold. Inexperienced users are advised to vomit if the need arises, as this social action loses none of the good stuff and does make the tripper feel considerably better.

Mescaline is almost always eaten, although it is possible to shoot, but the large quantities and side effects rule this out for all but the most determined needle freaks. The oral dose of mescaline is 300 to 500 milligrams (above 1 gram, toxic reactions may set in). Now, visualize a gram of coke, a pretty good sized pile, right? Now, figure 500 milligrams is half this size. This is the amount of real mescaline one must do in order to get off. ANY LESS THAN THIS, i.e., ANY PILLS OR CAPS THAT ARE LESS THAN HUGE ARE NOT MESCALINE. Simple as that, it is just not mescaline. It cannot be liquified and dropped on tablets, nor compressed into aspirin-sized pills.

Mescaline is a popular "in" drug, so pushers capitalize on this and sell just about anything as real mescaline. Normally, one can find every sort of LSD and a few LSD/PCP combinations being pushed as mescaline, and occasoinally much weirder things. . .Figure about, maybe five or six hits out of every one thousand are real mescaline.

Organic mescaline is a brown color with an earthy taste, synthetic is white crystal. Many less-than-scrupulously-honest pushers will dye acid brown or mix it with chocolate to get the appearance of mescaline.

Mescaline belongs to the amine group of chemicals (along with speed, STP, and several bodily drugs like adrenalin) it seems to effect both the mind and the body. All in all, it is a gentler trip than LSD, with less potential for a bummer. Users often experience a heightening of colors, sounds, and smells, but actual, out-and-out, comin'-off-the-wall hallucinations are rare. It seems to impart a champagne like bubbly, euphoric feeling and allows the user to maintain a seminormal expression and general attitude.

Tolerance does develop, although at a slower rate than with LSD, and cross-tolerance to both LSD and psilocybin does also develop.

The mescaline "trip" takes longer to come on than LSD, up to two hours, and seems to last about eight to ten hours. The crash is easier than the acid crash and the peak much less severe.

It is classified in the same category as LSD, and users/sellers/religious practitioners can expect the same penalities as those apprehended with acid can.

THE GREAT PEYOTE TRIP

It was in '69, I believe. We were operating an acid lab out of Boulder, Colorado, the new mecca for the unhooked generation. . . Three of our dealers and one chemist, who lived in North Carolina, of all places, had come to visit the U. of Colorado for a bash through summer school with a side of mixing and dealing. . .

We were getting pretty tired of acid as a steady diet and really sorta' dug mescaline from an aesthetic point of view. That is to say, it seemed to be more fun. Mescaline sulfate was just here and there, most of which had been made right in the University's science labs, so much, in fact, that the Boulder Feds were reported to have an open-dated warrant for the entire science department. A large MDA lab had just opened up, and as MDA was not too widely known and loved, it was usually getting the fake mescaline or psilocybin treatment.

John had run across a freak who claimed to have dug peyote in New Mexico, in full view of the highway. Fields and fields, he kept mumbling with a faraway look in his semiglazed eyes. He claimed to have waved to a highway patrol cruiser while he was busy digging, ever digging.

New Mexico, far out, right across the Rio Grande. Four of us rented a Hertz rent-a-van, and after carefully disconnecting the speedometer at the transmission to lighten the mileage, threw in the sleeping bags and split for the N.M. border.

We had all agreed to split the driving, but Sandy, one N.C. dealer, promptly conked out and slept through the better part of three states and two days. Crashed, just crashed.

Got down to N.M. and started looking for the proverbial yellow brick road. Nothing, man, one solid day of trucking around national parks and farmers fields. Ever tried to ask someone for a peyote field in N.M.? Ever tried to find someone you would ask for a peyote field in N.M.???

Blank. Nothing. Split for Arizona after checking the library in Rio something or other, where John deftly razored out the picture of the peyote cactus and the map showing its habitat.

Another day wandering around the burning sands of Arizona, carrying these fucking empty duffel bags to stash our find. . . One dried-up little, shriveled peyote cactus, man, the encyclopedia said they grew in fields — lies. . . all lies.

Dejected, eaten alive at Howard Johnson's, we head back up through N.M. to Colorado. Everybody is getting the downs. Four days of living in an unpadded Hertz rent-a-van, can bug anyone. . .everyone getting tired — no one wanting to drive. ..

Pete has eaten the one fucking dried-up little button. Shit, we don't even have any treasure now.

Someone suggests that we pool the stash and take some acid to awaken the spirit and the soul, as well as keep us awake for driving. Everyone drops a chocolate acid cap. . .about one hour later, three happy-go-lucky, stoned freaks and me. Nothing, man, nothing. . .watching the hills rush by and listening to the stoned riff — better take another cap. . .another half hour and I haven't gotten off, getting paranoid. . .what's the matter, can my tolerance be that high?. . .take the last identifiable pill in the stash — remainder is one funny white tablet. . .everyone hassling me, still no reaction. . .take the last unidentifiable little white tablet and jean pocket lint trip against everyone's advice. . . still not getting off.

We pull into a hick stop for gas. . .someone says, "I have heard that motion affects some people. You better watch it when you get out. . . "Bull-shit" . . . everyone hops out and heads for the munchies bar. "Fill 'er up," I tell the cowboy and open the door and RUSH. Everything is swirling around, can't stand, rushes going up and down my back with an incredible speed. . .my teeth raking out of my mouth. . .FLASH.

"What's a matter with you buddy. . ." Cowboy is drunk on his ass and looks unfriendly. . ."Far out, man," is all I can manage, sounds echo like I'm in the bottom of the well. . .standing at the Coke machine for I don't know how long. . .machine won't seem to take my money. Here comes the bad-ass cowboy. . .

"Hey, whatta ya trying to do to that machine?" Fuck. Can't seem to get the words out. "Ah, it won't eat my money, man. . ." Quarters spilling all over the ground. . .people pulling me back into the truck. . .wow, watch it man, yer blowing it. . .shit, keep it cool. . .just what I need to help reinforce the fact that I am too far-out fucking stoned. . .

Driving again. . .I told you not to take all that acid man, you gonna freak out. . .a friend in need. . .Pete is getting green, saying the peyote button is making him sick. . .Sandy, who has not said over two four-word sentences on this whole trip, is driving with an unhealthy concentration. I am in the lone passengers seat. . .

I start a running dialogue of a Gran Prix race. . .fine, you're doing fine, Sandy. . .we're almost in second place, now. This old Ferrari can really kick it in there man. . .Sandy is leaning over the wheel with a strange glow in his glazed eyes. . .OH, that son-of-a-bitch, Porsche captain has stuck a shill in front of us to hold us back. . .take him, man, you can take him. . .Sandy careening around corners on two wheels. We're on a little two-lane mountain road on the wrong side to pass the now panic-stricken Chevy in front of us, mumbling, "gonna win". . ."gotta win". . .I am hysterical. . .John and Pete are in the back frantically trying to open the back door, I think to jump. . .shut up, man. . . he's gonna kill us. . .make him slow down. . .

Now, down on a flat highway. . .it's dark. . .rushing along at top speed, about 90 miles per. . .Sandy has hunched completely over the wheel and is breathing heavily. . .I reach over and turn off the light switch. . .Suddenly, it is too dark, pitch dark with no sound and a freaky suspension of time and space. . .no movement sensation at all. . .we all look out into the strange darkness and suddenly, we can see the side posts shuttling past at a fantastic speed. . .all our collective hearts suddenly RUSH. I mean, a body rush that makes amyl nitrate look TAME. . .POUND, POUND everyone is frozen. CHRIST, whatta rush. . .John screams and jumps for the light switch. . .

Pete is moaning, stop. . .gonna be sick. . .John says to stop. . .Sandy, do you want to win this fucking race? No stops, Sandy mutters. . .I can hear the back door fly open as we hurtle around the next corner and hear Pete retching out into the 90 mph slipstream. . .Gonna win, mutters Sandy. . .whipping by a real Porsche. . .

Stop in Taos for a hamburger at an A & W. . .A real A & W, dig it. Four people so stoned that they can't talk, pulling into this A & W in a rented hippie van with a gold Hertz emblem. . .the only way to pry Sandy from the wheel was to pick up the monologue and convince him we had a pit stop. . .

Everyone gets the collective munchies. . .I want a hamburger and a cheeseburger and three onion rings and a mama burger and a shake. . .here, here man, you gotta order. . .we can't, too stoned. . .we'll blow it, man. . .get arrested in this cowboy town and hung. . .here, hundreds of dollar bills shoved at me in a fit of laughing paranoia. . .right, uh, uh. . .

About this time, I become aware of this strange metallic voice emanating out of blank space off to my left. Look out to see this pole with a speaker on it, "Can I help you. . .YOUR ORDER PLEASE". . .order. . .sure. "Uh, three cheeseburgers and four onion rings and one papa burger and three shakes and no, make that two cheeseburgers and two papa burgers and two root beers instead of the shakes and two hot fudge sundaes and just three orders of onion". . .eevryone is hassling me and I'm trying to repeat the orders as fast as they come in. . .the damn machine has now taken on the characteristics of a robot and is sounding angrier and angrier. . .I can't possibly keep up with all that. I have always had this deep-rooted psychological fear of machines taking over the world, anyway, and now I can suddenly visualize the problems. . .all coming to a head with this machine that has the gall to order me around. . .

Next thing I remember, I am leaning out of the driver's seat and strangling the pole with my hands, really getting into shaking it back and forth. . .screaming God Damn robot, take that, you so and so. . .the other three freaks trying to pull me back into the van. . .suddenly we look up right into a dead silence. . . rows of '57 freaks in those jacked-up Chevys staring at us with these incredibly disbelieving looks. . .I am yanked back into the van and someone sits in the driver's seat. . .tearing out of the parking lot amidst much swearing and confusion. . .I still have several wires in my clenched fist. . .

Stoned, but pressing on into the night, gradually everyone starts crashing badly, four days of travel and the night's excitement combined with the natural down time of the acid, and they are drifting out of it. Here, you drive. . . I am still stoned and talking a blue streak to three lifeless bodies. . .everyone is asleep and I am wired from coming on so much later than everyone else. . . tracers on all the headlights. . .up into Colorado, I began crashing. . .prying my eyes open through sheer will power. . .trucking on. . .some sort of psychedelic patterns swirling around me over and over, red flashes. . .SHIT, it's the pigs, pull over man. . .

Badge. . .Stiff face. . .Been following you for ten miles with the light on. . .Oh yeah, sorry, thought you were after someone else. . .Wow, you guys look out of it. . .yeah, sure, ticket written, too tired to be paranoid. . .back driving. . .through Denver. . .we creep into Boulder as utter failures before the first light of dawn. . .

MORPHINE

Morphine is an alkaloid occurring naturally in opium. Morphine is about 1/10th the weight of opium. It was isolated and used in the Orient as a cure for opium addiction. Needless to say. . .

Morphine is an excellent pain-killer and is still used in medicine for that purpose. The drug's other effects include a feeling of general lethargy, loss of hunger and sex drive, flushing of the skin, and a general feeling of euphoria.

It is taken orally or by injection. The oral method decreases its potent effect somewhat, but tends to make the overall high last longer.

Tolerance does appear after a time of steady use and can necessitate huge doses to get any effect at all.

Pure morphine is really not soluble in water, so normal medical and street morphine is usually in the form of morphine sulfate, which is readily soluble in water. It is habit forming and produces severe withdrawal symptoms.

Morphine is an upper class drug because of limited access. Most users in the U.S. are doctors, pharmacists, clinical workers, or others with medical availability. Street morphine is rare; most ends up as smack.

MYRISTICA OIL

This is the active constituent of nutmeg and can still be occasionally purchased. Myristica oil contains about 4 per cent MMDA.

It can be consumed as is (a bit much for the stomach, as it is a smelly, super oily oil), or the MMDA can be distilled out by steam distillation.

OPIUM

Opium is extracted from the unripe seed pods of a far eastern poppy (Papaver sonniferum) and dried to form a dark brown, gummy substance. Opium smoking became very popular in China in the 1800's, so much so, that the government attempted to outlaw its use and import. This proposed law caused Britain to go to war against China (as Britain was making money importing the opium into China). Needless to say, Britain won, and millions of Chinese became opium addicts.

In the 1800's, opium was offered in many over-the-counter cough syrups and general tonics in America. By the end of the century, an estimated one in every 400 Americans was addicted to opium. The major group of addicts was housewives who used the addictive mixtures to combat the boredom of housekeeping. This fact may be the primary reason that it took so long to start Women's Lib.

Opium is normally smoked by heating it in a water pipe (it does not burn well by itself, but rather tends to vaporize) or, as practiced by American freaks heated by the application of a hot knife blade or soldering iron and the resulting vapor inhaled through a drinking straw.

Opium addiction is rare in the U.S. In fact, it is seldom we find any real opium on the streets (although several types of incense resemble it closely, and we DO find this on the streets) because opium can be converted to the much more profitable states of morphine and heroin.

An opium stone is a drugged, heavy feeling, wherein the user often wants to just sit there and do nothing except smoke. It often causes some nausea in inexperienced users.

Users do develop a tremendous tolerance level and must take larger and larger doses (up to 20 - 40 grams a day) to get off. Overdoses are possible (especially when shooting), but the level varies because heavy addicts can just get off on a dosage which might kill a nonaddict.

PCP

Phencyclidine (PCP) is a legit drug manufactured under the trade name of Sernyl from Parke-Davis. It is commonly used as a tranquilizer and an anesthetic for animals in veterinary situations.

It is marked alone as THC, Angels Dust (usually sprayed on mint leaves), Hog, Peace Pills, and Rhino or animal trank.

PCP is occasionally mixed with other drugs, notably acid, to produce a different reaction. The dealer can pawn it off on the buyer as mescaline or psilocybin, as these drugs are more popular than acid and bring a better price.

General nervous system effects of PCP are numbness, sedation, anesthesia. It can also cause muscle incoordination, double vision, and dizziness.

For some reason, PCP seems to cause an unusually high preoccupation with death in users. It can also cause changes in bodily awareness such as a feeling of diminishing size.

Disassociation of the hands and legs is common, as is a tingling sensation all over the body.

The worst application seems to be on mint or parsley sold as "Superweed," or "Angel's Dust." Lighting up a joint of what is expected to be righteous weed and finding yourself in a full-blown PCP trip, which resembles a hallucinogenic drug, not unlike DMT, may be a shock for the unwary. It can also amplify latent tendencies and psychoses such as acid is prone to do.

The effects of PCP usually wear off in about four hours.

PCP was once used as a human tranquilizer, but given up after a number of people experienced bad side effects. It first appeared on the street scene in the summer of '67 as a "Peace Pill." This pill gave moderate effects, but tended to produce bummers when taken in conjunction with other drugs. It disappeared to resurface as THC.

Poorly made PCP can cause convulsions, coughing up, and other bad reactions. The drug combines badly with alcohol and may cause death in the manner of reds and alcohol.

The major result of PCP intake is a feeling of weedlike euphoria which is usually enjoyable. The problem is that it mixes badly with most other drugs and increased dosages, or even repeated use of just PCP, can cause a speedlike paranoia. PCP does have a definite overdose potential and can be physically addictive, but not as heavily as Sopors, smack or reds.

When PCP is smoked, a noticeable chemical smell tends to remain in the air.

PSILOCYBIN AND MUSHROOMS

Psilocybin is one of the active ingredients of the Mexican sacred mushroom, Psilocybin mexicana, which frequents the Yucatan Peninsula, but does not extend into the U.S. It is also found in several varieties of other psilocybe mushrooms which can be found in the U.S.

Synthetic psilocybin has been successfully produced in a number of "underground" attempts, BUT shares the same drawbacks as synthetic mescaline; i.e. difficult to manufacture, expensive, and no where NEARLY as profitable to make as good ol' LSD. So, as one might surmise, there is very, very little real psilocybin floating around the streets.

The demand for psilocybin is high. Real, honest-to-God psilocybin, produces a nice controlled high, which is not as disorienting as acid. As the dosage increases, it reaches the hallucinogenic stage and becomes "spiritual" in feeling. It is more potent than mescaline, and, hence, carries a greater bad trip risk.

A normal dose of psilocybin is 14 - 40 milligrams which yields about a six hour trip, but the length does increase with the dosage. It brings on the classic symptoms of nausea as does mescaline, and, as with mescaline, these are more prevalent in the organic versions than in the synthetics.

The magic ingredient in psilocybin is a phosphoric ester of 4-hydroxydimethytryptamine. It contains the same indole ring as LSD

On a street level, about one in every 1,000 doses of purported psilocybin is really psilocybin. The others are the usual weak acid or acid-PCP combinations.

A new trip is to spike mushrooms (the common store variety) with LSD and sell them as psilocybin. A look at the relative dosages and identifying features should quickly allow the user to tell the difference.

Occasionally, dried mushrooms hit the streets. This makes the visual ID difficult, if not impossible, so look at your source. Would you eat a specialized, difficult-to-find substance from this guy? Consider it.

There are over 15 different varieties of the psilocybin mushroom. Some three or four of these species occur naturally in the United States, primarily in the south. These mushrooms all contain the active alkaloids psylibin and psilocyin, and each gives about the same response in the body.

Any of the mushrooms may be dried at room temperature and kept potent for years.

The commonest psilocybin mushroom species in this country are: Psilocybe cubensis, Panaeolus subbalteatus, and Psilocybe caerulescens. The most common of these three is Psilocybe cubensis.

Finding the mushrooms is a relatively easy task for anyone in the correct locale. The psilocybe family grows ONLY: A. In the southern part of the U.S., except the psilocybe cubensis, which has been found just about everywhere from northern California on down. B. It grows only on manure (cow, pig, goat, etc.) C. And in the months where the temperature ranges between 65 - 85 degrees.

Identifying the mushrooms is only slightly harder. HOWEVER, the novice should not eat any mushroom in the field and should only nibble a tiny bite of any fungi brought back to the house, and only those which passed the tests for appearance and psilocybin alkaloid.

Any psilocybin mushroom will turn a distinctive bluish tint when bruised or broken and left alone for twenty minutes to one hour. The bluish bruise is an indication of the active alkaloid and will appear first on the inside of the broken stem. Another positive test is described in the TESTING section of this book. (There is one non psilocybin species which gives the characteristic bluish tint, but it differs radically in physical appearance.)

The "mushroom" part of the plant is actually the fruit which grows underneath the ground for some time and then comes through the soil when the conditions are just right. This fruit matures quite fast and a difference of a couple of hours can mean a difference in appearance.

Psilocybe cubensis: The cap is about ½" to 4" across and switches from a conical shape (in the first few hours of life) to a convex and then to a flat shape with the edges upraised slightly. The color can vary from white with a gold center circle to light brown (still with the gold center).

If it absorbs an abundance of water, the cap will become clear and the blue-olive spores will show through. When any color is dried, it will go to a yellow-brown and still have the gold center circle.

The gills range from a light brown when young to a deep purple or black when mature.

The stem will range from 1" to 6" tall, hollow, and have a lighter tint than the cap.

The meat has little color and tastes a bit like grain. It is found on manure or soil that has a high manure content.

Panaeolus subbalteatus: The cap will be cone shaped and usually light brown in color. In the younger stages, it will be colored by light flecks. In young fungi, there is a white veil that hangs down, but disappears with age.

The gills are light brown to black depending on age and are closely spaced.

The stem ranges from 1" to 4" and is seldom over ½" thick. The lower portion of the stem is covered with a sheet of small scales and a white powder. The stem is hollow and usually white or just off-white.

It is not as common as psilocybe cubensis, but frequents the same haunts, so to speak.

Psilocybe Caerulescens: The cap is between 1" and 3" across and also goes from the cone shape when young, to the flat or convex shape as it grows up. The surface of the cap is smooth and sticky and translucent when wet. In older fungi, the margins will be a different shade than the center and appear in a ring shape, while in youngsters, the color is a green to black. This separation of color rings is usually irregular in shape.

The gills are close together, light brown, which darkens with age.

The stem is 1" to 4" tall and up to ½" thick. It is hollow and smooth and its top, with thick hairs running up the rest of the stem. The stem is quite tough.

The meat is off-white to yellow with a strong grainlike odor. This species can occasionally be found in moist swamps or riverbanks in the southern United States.

EXTRACTION

One can extract the magic ingredients of any psilocybin mushroom by drying the mushrooms and grinding them into a powder. The psilocybin is then extracted by soaking in methyl alcohol for a couple of days and letting the clear fluid evaporate in a flat dish for several days. The residue can be resoaked/evaporated for more concentration.

However, there is no harm in just eating the mushroom as it. A normal dose is about four to six of the American varieties. The trip is not unlike a cross between grass and mescaline, with the grasslike high and mescaline body rush and color intensities.

Amanita muscaria: This is the mushroom usually referred to as the sacred mushroom of the Mexican and Aztec cultures and used by the Russians and several other primitive tribes. It is not a psilocybin mushroom, but rather, contains a hallucinogenic drug called muscarin, which is related to belladonna and can be nullified by atropine. There is much controversy surrounding the use of Amanita muscaria, some anthropologists have declared it a poison of the killing order, while many heads and some reliable sources say the poison resembles the poisoning of mescaline.

At any rate, Amanita muscaria grows in Mexico as well as California, Michigan, Wisconsin, and Minnesota. If you are going to experiment, BE SURE of your ID and try small quantities ONLY. The following recipe seems to be one that has been kicking around for some time as to the preparation of this mushroom and MAY alleviate any toxic effects.

Collect about 20 - 25 medium-sized mushrooms and wash them to remove dirt and other impurities. Chop them into small pieces and lay them on tin foil or a cookie sheet. Put into a preheated oven of 225 - 250 degrees (NO MORE THAN 250) with the door open a bit. Let cook for about five - six hours, the pieces should be very dry and crumbly, then smash into a fine powder.

This powder may be taken straight or mixed with other foods. A normal dosage is about five - eight teaspoonsfuls (or about three-four mushrooms).

Identification: The Amanita muscaria is variable in several departments; the cap ranges from white to brown to blood red. Pieces of veil are scattered around the outer surface and resemble cottage cheese. It has a large bulb, which resembles a puffball, and a short stem.

One of the problems here is that a couple of close cousins to Amanita muscaria are very definitely poisonous, usually to a fatal extent: Neither cousin resembles the Amanita muscaria too closely. The danger lies in the fact that someone decides it's a close enough relative to have some psychedelic redeeming value.

These relatives are: Amanita virosa (Destroying Angel), Amanita verna, and Amanita phalloides (Death Cup). In appearance, these fungi are tall and vary from white to gray-brown to green, usually, they will have wartlike patches, which can be easily removed, on the caps. All have a bulb on the base of the stem. The Amanita Phalloides will bruise reddish-brown when damaged.

If you are interested in further information on American sources of psilocybin (including growing your own), send your name to: Guidance Publications, P.O. Box 15667, New Orleans, Louisiana 70175, and ask to be put on their mailing list.

Good reference books for the prospective hunter are: Field-

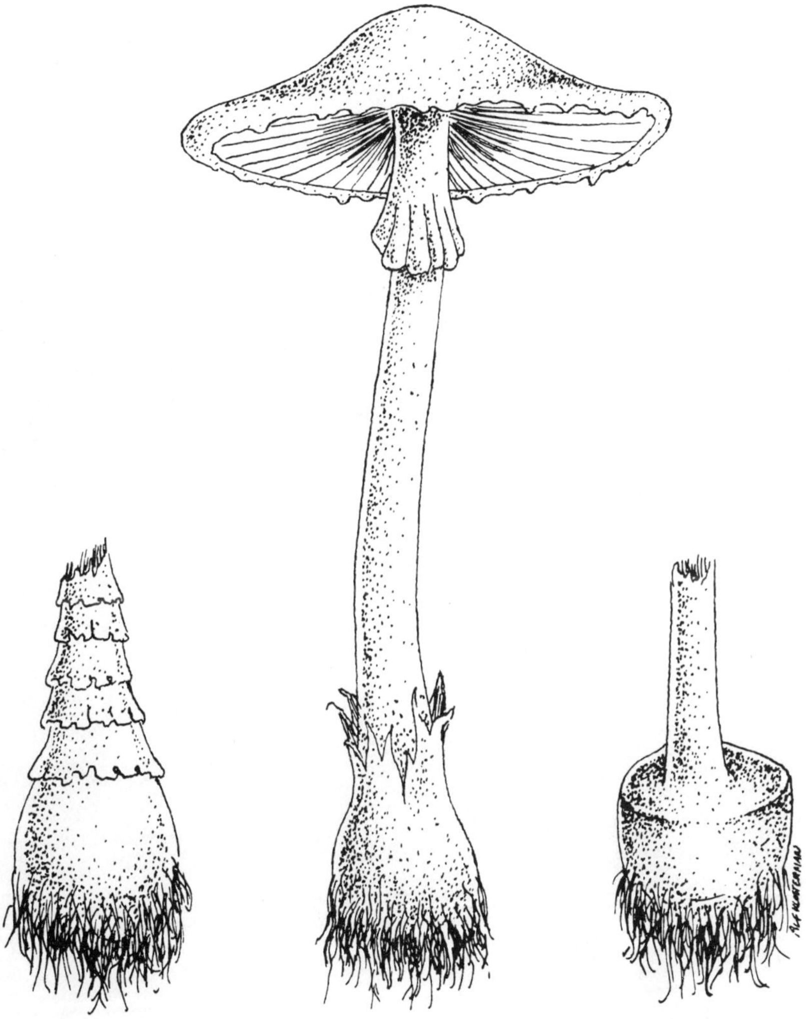

A. muscaria A. virosa A. mappa

The highly poisonous "Death Cup and Destroying Angel," members of the Amanita family sometimes confused with psychotropic cousins. All can be recognized by the bulb at the base of the stem.

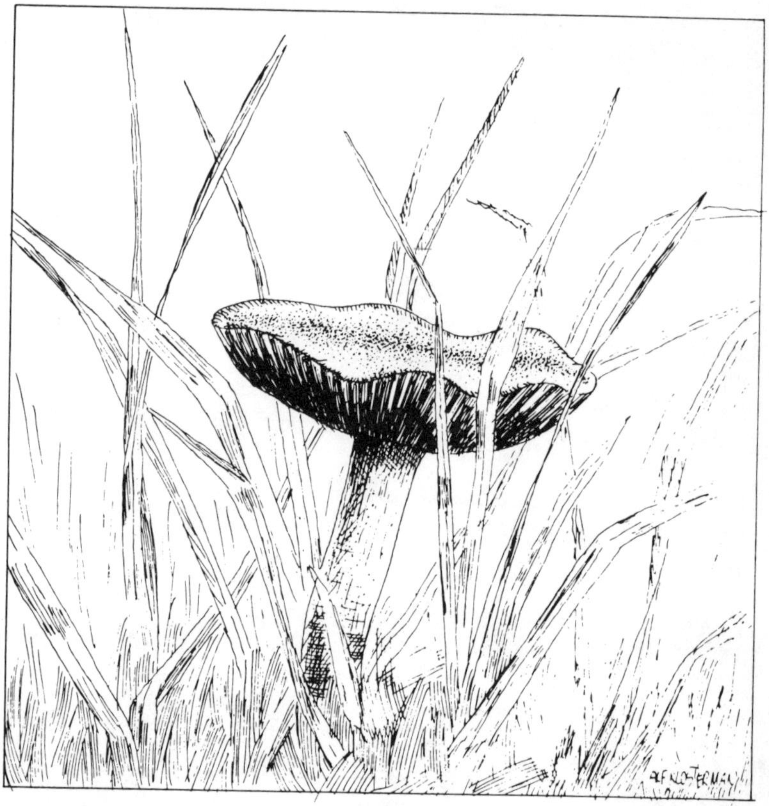

Psilocybe cubensis – A "common" North American psychotropic fungi.

book of Common Mushrooms, Sturgis, G.P. Putnam and Sons, New York; and Mushroom Hunters' Field Guide, Smith, University of Michigan Press, Ann Arbor, Michigan.

Another hallucinogenic mushroom is Amanita muscaris. This mushroom grows wild in the midwestern part of the U.S. and is becoming increasingly available on the drug market.

It is listed as a poison in several accounts, but other cultures do use it in rites and such, and the poisoning seems to be on the same order as the poisoning a peyote button gives you. HOWEVER, this is not guaranteed, you know, you are taking a bit of a risk.

WHEN YOU USE ANY MUSHROOM, GET A COPY OF A GUIDE TO MUSHROOMS AND TOADSTOOLS OR DICTIONARY OF FUNGI AND BE POSITIVE OF YOUR ID – THE GUY WHO TURNED YOU ONTO IT MAY NOT KNOW AS MUCH AS HE CLAIMS.

QUAALUDE

Quaalude, or by its correct name, methaqualone, (or by its correcter name, 2-Methyl-3-ortho-tolyl-4-quinazolone) is a non-barbiturate drug, which produces a sedative, hypnotic state similar to barbiturates. Quaalude is a glutethemide drug (along with Doriden and Methyproglon) and is prescribed for insomnia and preoperative sedation.

Quaalude is listed (at the time of this writing) in the Physician's Desk Reference as a nonaddictive sedative with only minor cautionings about prescribing. Consequently, a lot of doctors have been prescribing it instead of a barb. The FDA has Quaalude in a fairly minor category of scheduled drugs (again, at the time of this writing), but seems about to classify it as a Schedule 2 drug, along with such things as amphetamine, methadone, coke, etc.

Quaalude develops a relaxed down "high," wherein the user is still able to function at a passable level. It doesn't produce the low emotional reactions of reds, although a distinct lack of coordination begins to take effect at moderate dosages, and a lack of memory is quite pronounced in heavy users.

Quaalude was pitched as an aphrodisiac for some time. In actuality, it does release inhibitions, to about the same effect as two Margarita's. It drops the tripper into a relaxed, loose mood, and allows pleasant sex, although in moderate to heavy doses, it has the same effect on the male as heavy alcohol does. That is to say, it make it rough.

It is a pleasant high with little drug hangover and is fairly inexpensive due to the generosity of the drug companies in manufacturing such large quantities. This all adds up to the ease in which one may cop a Quaalude attitude, much the same as drinking. Pop a couple to wake up with, pop a couple before lunch, pop a couple before going out.

The problem is that Quaalude is not only psychologically addictive, but extremely physically addictive. A user can develop physical withdrawal symptoms in as little as one month of eight to ten Quaaludes a day.

The withdrawal symptoms are similar to smack, flulike running of the nose, cramps, stomach trouble, etc. True withdrawal takes on the characteristics of barbiturate withdrawal (which is WORSE than heroin withdrawal), grand mal convulsions, delirium, mania, dizziness, stomach hemorrhaging and other such pleasantries.

To compound the problem, it is much harder to cure Quaalude addiction than even barb addiction. The only "safe" method in heavy cases is hospitalization and total abstinence from Quaalude while substituting barbiturates. When one is addicted to the barbs instead of the Quaalude, the doctors can treat for barb addiction.

Some people are attempting to shoot Quaalude. Not good. Very alkaline and very likely to cause abscesses and cellulitis.

Heavy lude freaks can be recognized, much as heavy speed freaks can. They have an inability to cope with normal situations and people. A heavy lude user acts much like a lobotomy patient; lets his head roll from side to side, repeats the same sentences over and over, no motivation except to remember to feed the habit.

Another problem is drug interreaction. Quaalude is absorbed by the intestine at an irregular rate and reacts heavily with other drugs and alcohol. It is possible to take two or three ludes and drink and wind up with a heavy overdose. NEVER MIX DOWNERS WITH EACH OTHER OR ALCOHOL.

If you are hot to try lude, take it very easy the first few times. Take a small dose, stay loose. Never keep around more than you plan to take, as people have gotten confused and forgotten how many they've done and used too many during the course of the trip.

By itself, Quaalude reaches the acute OD stage at about 2.4 grams (about 8 - 300 mg. tabs) with coma and convulsions (and the possibility of choking to death on your vomit a la Jimi Hendrix) and death at 3 grams.

Because of the nonexistent possibility of a bad trip, and the other various attractions, Quaalude use is still on the definite upswing. On the East Coast, there are "fruit bars," that deal to lude freaks who come in and drink fruit juice and groove to down music. Quaalude is big for parties because of the relaxed, no hassle atmosphere it imparts, and a whole "culture" is growing up around lude, much as the grass and acid cultures did.

Oddly enough, Quaaulde is somewhat of a regional drug, more popular in the Midwest and East than in the drug centers of the West Coast. Each particular brand seems to be found (hmmmmm. . .) in heavy concentrations around its manufacturers, i.e.: Rorer (Quaalude) is in Philadelphia, and oddly enough, Philly is swamped with Quaalude; Wallace in New Jersey makes Optimil and New Jersey has an Optimil problem; Parke-Davis in Detroit does Parest and Detroit is covered with Parest; Sopor made in Illinois by Arnar-Stone is big in Chicago and the Midwest. ...

All in all, it is a shit drug. Nice in small quantities, but too easy to get into and too rough to get out of.

IDENTIFICATION:

Quaalude — Rorer — 150 mgs (white) — 300 mgs (white) — 500 mgs (white)

Sopor — Anar-Stone — 75 mgs (green) — 150 mgs (yellow) — 300 mgs (orange) all with A/S on pills

Optimil — Wallace — 200 mgs and 400 mgs in blue or pink cpas

Somnafac — Smith, Miller and Patch — 200 mgs in two-tone blue caps, 400 mgs (Fourte) in dark blue caps

Parest — Parke-Davis — 200 mgs and 400 mgs in pink or blue caps

Biphetamine — Strasenburgh — Biphetamine T 12½ 6.25 mgs amphetamine, 6.25 dex, 40 mgs lude

Biphetamine 20 — 10 mgs of each amphetamine with same Quaalude.

Several times, when we had run dry of lysergic acid, we made speed. A soul kitchen took less skill and the profit was still good. P_2P was fairly easy to get in those days, so, we would whip up a batch.

A couple of incidents convinced me that I didn't want to shoot speed. Every now and again, I had the privilege of tasting the speed after every batch. This meant an oral tasting, as the speed was too wet with ether to shoot. Wet speed tastes like eating a sweet tart made from ether. It literally explodes all over your taste buds, and the doctor's office mouth stays with you for several hours afterwards. . .

When the speed had dried (under a sunlamp), we would have to find a volunteer to test it. We even had a fit, just for this use.

One time, we dug up this freak who had been doing speed for several years. "Hey, man, want to do us a favor? We need someone to test this speed to see how good it is. . ."

The guy couldn't believe it, you know, he kept trying to figure out what the catch was. "Sure, I'll help"

We took him into an apartment and sat him on the edge of the bathtub where he cooked up about an eighth of a teaspoon.

"Ahh, don't you think that's a bit heavy. . ." I said.

"Shit, man, I can do up a whole fucking spoon if I really want to get off."

"Yeah, but this is pure speed, I mean, it's not cut with anything. You better take it easy."

"All the stuff I get is pure, man. I don't do any cut shit." He stuck the needle in his arm, squeezed, and hung there suspended for a minute with this incredulous look on his face, then he stuttered something like, "Goddddddddd" and fell over on his head in the bathtub, quivering all over.

We hauled him back up and he was so wired that he couldn't move. Wired, literally stiff. We slapped his face and helped him maintain, figuring he was about to die, you know. Finally, he gets it together enough to talk.

We all look down and see the needle is still stuck in his arm. . ."Shit, MAN, can I do up some more of that stuff?"

The other time was when a doctor sold me 2,000 of these whites that he claimed were about 15 per cent pure meth. I wandered around San Francisco, which was just about flat dried up for crystal, until I found this freak friend. "You know anybody who can try this stuff and give me a good report?"

His eyes widened, "yeah. . ."

We ended up in a speed house. Four or five freaks, all bosom buddies lived there and did up speed. They had been flat out for about four days and were around in circles muttering, "When is that muther going to be back with that ounce?" "Man, I can't go on much longer," and other encouraging epitaphs. No one took any notice of me, so I held out my fist and said, "Would anyone try this speed and see how good it is?"

There was a stunned silence and suddenly I had four people grabbing my hand, forcing it open. These bosom buddies were like really hitting each other in the face trying to get the pills. . .shit, gimme one, come on. . .finally, we got it organized and I said "Don't shoot it, I've heard a French Chalk base can make you go blind if you shoot. . .just drop them."

Next thing I knew, someone was cooking them up with a little water, "NAW, we'll just shoot the top layer and not get any base, who cares, if you gotta go, you gotta go". . .And these freaks shot my little ten-cent-apiece pills, risking their eyes without so much as a second thought. . .

FRANK ZAPPA ONCE SAID, "I WOULD SUGGEST YOU DON'T USE SPEED, AND HERE'S WHY: IT WILL MESS UP YOUR LIVER, YOUR KIDNEYS, ROT YOUR MIND. IN GENERAL, THIS DRUG WILL MAKE YOU JUST LIKE YOUR MOTHER AND FATHER."

SPEED

Speed refers to any drug with an amphetamine base, including: Amphetamines (Benzedrine), methamphetamine (Methedrine, Desoxyn, Amphedroxyn, Norodin, etc.), Dextroamphetamines (Dexedrine, Dexamyl), and so on.

When we refer to speed in a street sense, we are usually talking about meth, or methamphetamine hydrochloride, in a crystal form.

Speed, in all forms, is a central nervous system stimulant, which acts in ways similar to the body's own epinephrine (like adrenalin). It works by increasing the concentrations of the chemical that makes the connections between nerve cells. This greatly stimulates the bodily processes.

Until very recently, over 20 per cent of all the prescriptions written in the U.S. were for one form of speed or another. This should give you some sort of clue to our lifestyle.

Most of the speed in tablet form is amphetamine sulfate. The most common varieties are the mini-white pills with crosses etched upon them, scoring the tab into four equal parts. Mini-whites started out on a medical basis and are now almost strictly bootleg. Much of the street supply in this country comes from Mexico, although some is made in the U.S.

Mini-whites seem to test out very pure, BUT out of several batches of identical mini-whites tested, the dosage varied from 2.5 mg to 10 mg. This situation creates a very real danger in the fact that one can become used to downing a handful of weak mini-whites and then unknowingly swallow an equal number of superpotent tablets, creating an overdose potential.

Another form of amphetamine sulfate is Benzedrine, which comes in rose-colored heart-shaped tabs or oval shaped footballs.

Physical dependence on speed does not occur in the normal

definition of the term. However, chronic use of the drug leads to a buildup of excitability or lack of fatigue, which turns into manic depression, tremors, muscle twitches, etc., when the user is away from the drug, which, of course, makes it easy to hit it up again.

Crystal can be snorted, eaten, or injected. The taste of speed is a harsh chemical, and very few people continue to eat it for long.

The normal method of use is by injection. Speed produces an orgasmiclike rush moments after entering the bloodstream. Many users will shoot more than necessary to maintain the high, just to re-experience this flash.

Tolerance does occur in great amounts, forcing the user to consume large quantities to get off at all.

Occasionally, users will mix barbiturates with speed to help remove the paranoid nervousness of the speed and alleviate the barbiturate hangover. This combination can lead to an unknown barbiturate addiction in the heavy user.

A commercial type of downer-upper is Dexamyl, a combination of amphetamine sulfate and amobarbital.

THE TRIP

After the initial rush, speed produces a great feeling of well-being and elation, as well as a feeling of unlimited power.

The pupils dilate, you sweat, your heart is greatly speeded up, and your mucous membranes dry up. (This side effect of speed has been put to great use in the nasal inhalers which, until recently, contained Benzedrine. A hard-up user could smash the inhaler, soak the cotton in water, and shoot up the works. This lead to abscesses, burns, heat rashes, and other fun things).

The user tends to become very talkative and his interest span increases greatly. He is often able to concentrate on one thing to the exclusion of all else. (One of the people helping with this book spent his first speed "trip" watching a free movie on spark plugs at an airport, over and over and over.) This ability to concentrate is often valued by students who do up a large hit to cram for tests.

A person's IQ may actually increase several points while on speed, but whatever he absorbs tends to be lost in the shuffle of the crash.

The feeling of very well-being and power lasts throughout the trip, but is replaced by a period of being down after the trip is over.

The avoidance of this down time often encourages users to rehit as the first dose begins wearing off. This in turn leads to a "run," during which the user will stay up for as much as four to five days during which he doesn't eat or sleep much.

After this run, he falls into a deep sleep state for as much as 18 hours. After he awakens, he is famished, depressed, lethargic, and thinks what another hit would do for him.. . .

Weight loss can be as high as 25 pounds in one speed run, abscesses are common, skin ulcers appear, and teeth soon begin to drop out.

Speed activates the entire body and forces it to function at an abnormally high rate for a long period of time. This burns out the body. A heavy speed user can cram several years of aging into a few short months. It lowers the body's resistance to disease as well as gradually destroys the user's memory

Vocabularies can decrease to a few hundred words (notably present are: "hey, man, wow, flash, rush, fucking, etc."), and sexual performance is impaired.

The old saying, notwithstanding, speed rarely kills, directly, at least. However, heroin addicts have a longer life expectancy than speed freaks. Ever know a speed freak who had been using heavily for ten years? Five? If so, he is a walking corpse. . .

Speed also has the interesting ability to cause heavy, unjustified paranoia. This paranoia is doubly exciting as you never know when it is going to strike, although, runs of several days seem to increase the chances at a square of rate.

USING

If you just gotta use speed, remember: It makes life difficult for the kidneys and liver, so drink lots of liquids. Food is not properly absorbed by the body when using, even if you force yourself to eat. Vitamins help compensate to some degree, especially the B complexes and C taken in high doses. Lots of milk or yogurt are good additions, as it tends to help if the body absorbs any remaining quantities of speed in the blood. The milk and yogurt also replace lost calcium.

If you have to come down in a hurry, Librium or Valium can help, and a Seconal will do it in an emergency, BUT avoid getting into this habit or a speed/red habit will soon develop.

Also, realize the heavy power trip speed brings about usually changes personalities. If you are withdrawn, you may find yourself speaking out more and more. If you are normally obnoxious, you will probably become quite unbearable. Friends have a way of disappearing, unless, of course, they are also speed freaks, but who would want speed freaks for friends?

Meth used to come from the widespread medical sources. As these gradually dried up, underground chemists began producing speed by converting Phenyl $_2$ *Proponone (*P_2P*) into crystal by oxidizing it with aluminum foil, salt, hydrochloric acid, water, ether, and alcohol. The mixture works for about six hours. Its ph is brought up to 7 by adding acid, and the whole mixture is boiled off in stages until only the liquified speed remains. Then it is dumped into stirred ether, where it crystalizes. The ether is then vacuum suctioned through ordinary filter paper, which leaves the speed.*

The speed is left to dry for at least twelve hours and then placed upon a mirror and chopped with a razor blade and forced through nylon stockings to "fluff" it up. It is cut, usually with talcum powder, quinine, epsom salts.

The process is not difficult and produces a high yield, somewhere on the order of a pound of speed per two pounds of P_2P*. Federal agents put a stop to* P_2P *sales, except under restricted conditions, which forced it to come in from Canada or England.*

P_2P *can be synthesized by a pressure fractional distillation method, but it is a difficult job, on a higher level than manufacturing speed.*

The whole process takes about 18 - 24 hours, and the boiling of the ether-alcohol-water-speed mixture produces a characteristic odor of a smelly doctor's office burning down. This means that your lab must be well ventilated (it is explosive), and the odor disguised, as any chemist and/or cop can sniff this a block away.

SPEED

A strange formula appeared in the 1800's for home brew speed. It appears to contain all the necessary chemical elements for meth, but we have never tried this and can definitely not guarantee that it would work or that the end product would even be safe to fool around with.

Place several pieces of SOFT coal in a bowl. In a separate bowl combine:

6 tablespoons salt

6 tablespoons Blue Boy or Rosebud bluing compound

6 tablespoons water

1 tablespoon of ammonia (concentrated)

Pour the mixture over the coal.

Crystals will begin to form soon after the materials are brought together and will continue to do so for several days. Every so often, add some more ammonia water to replace that which is consumed by the reaction.

STP

STP (or DOM, or 4-methyl-2,5-dimethoxy-a-methylphenethylamine) is one of the ideal situations in which freaks and private industry have cooperated.

STP was originally known as BZ and was a top secret nerve gas being developed for the Army by Dow Chemical Company. The idea behind this was that you could spray a town with BZ, walk in, and take over without firing a shot, as no one would really feel like fighting back, while in the throes of a deep hallucinogenic trip.

BZ was synthesized by a Dow chemist, and soon, maybe just days afterward, it was found to be floating around in hip society. This meant: A.) A gang of ruthless hippies had conspired, broken into the top secret Dow labs, sneaked past the guards, picked the safe which contained the formula, and sneaked out with it; or B.) Some straight, God-fearing, Dow chemist invented the drug, looked at his salary, looked at the tremendous market for LSD, and stole it, reselling to the "underground" chemists.

You choose.

STP resembles mescaline. That is, it is also an amphetamine-based drug. An STP trip lasts longer than an LSD trip, up to three or four days, and is more intense (although the drug is less potent than LSD on a per weight basis).

The psychotropic reaction experienced with STP is likened to a release of untapped energy, a feeling of being able to do anything, coupled with a feeling of not being able to stop. STP produces hallucinations but not as disoriented as LSD. You see the same things as when you're straight, must in a different sense.

The way to cope with an STP trip seems to be able to flow with the energy, not oppose it. The chances of bad tripping seem to be greatly increased with STP, as much as a possible 60/40 chance of a bummer.

STP first came to light in the summer of '67, when about ten bummers were reported to San Francisco hospitals in 11 days. STP was given out on a free basis at a "love in" in San Francisco, and many bummers resulted. This was complicated by the fact that tranquilizers, like those usually used to combat an LSD overdose (chlorpromazine, etc.) seem to intensify an STP trip if taken after the peak. (Although, they seem to calm it if taken before the peak.)

Most tabs of STP seem to contain about ten milligrams of the drug, a dose of only four milligrams will get one off. The larger the dose, the longer and more intense the trip is likely to be.

STRYCHNINE

A terribly misunderstood drug. Strychnine is almost nonexistent in street drugs. The strychnine rumors floating around are usually started because of two factors:

1. Strychnine does cause hallucinogenic reactions.

2. Overdoses of LSD cause identical symptoms as strychnine poisoning. This panics people with some knowledge of drugs into thinking their LSD is padded with strychnine for additional effect. It is almost, universally, not true.

Strychnine will cause convulsions and respiratory depression and possibly death, in amounts of 15-30 micrograms. Death usually occurs in 20 - 30 minutes.

THC

One thing first — THC does exist. HOWEVER, NOT ON THE STREET! ! ! Never. Never. THC would cost about $6 for the RAW chemicals (in the common synthesis), so figure about 1,000 per cent markup to hit the street, and we come out with $60 a hit. If you are buying $2 THC, IT IS NOT! Most likely, it is PCP.

THC was isolated in 1964, in Israel, in a process known as Delta 1. Since this time a Delta 6 process has also been isolated which contains the same active agents.

The complexity and cost of the raw chemicals in either of these methods (although the Delta 6 is a bit cheaper) prohibit the drug from reaching the street. However, recent almost-breakthroughs show the possibility of synthesizing cheap THC from essential organic oils found in lichens. This is not feasible on a major level due to the hassle and large beginning/little end product, but may someday be the answer to the average freak, who wants to try some real, honest-to god THC.

Another, although admittedly, temporary advantage to this process is the fact that the BNDD doesn't know about it yet.

The only practical method of obtaining "real" THC is by extraction and conversion from nature's own source, marijuana, as shown in the hash oil section.

This may be partially outdated in the near future, as an active synthesis has now been published, which could conceivably bring the cost of THC manufactured "grass" down to about $40 a kilo, but this is NOT being done at the present time, and is still a VERY complex process, so don't get excited.

Pure THC would be about twenty times as potent as good hash. Due to this fact, and the neat concept involved with THC, many pushers sell various other chemicals as THC. The most common bootleg THC is PCP, an animal tranquilizer, which is no longer given to humans due to bad side effects. Real THC must be stored in a cool place or it loses its potency.

OTHERS

Alphaprodine (Nisentil, Nisintil, Prisiliden) Synthetic drug related to morphine, although a bit weaker. Habit forming.

Amyl Nitrate – (Poppers, Snappers). Inhaled to dilate the blood vessels during a heart attack. Produces a temporary, superspeedy effect.

Amytal – Hypnotic barbiturate. (Lilly – green – 15 milligrams, yellow – 30, orange – 50, pink – 100.)

Amytal Sodium – Heavy barbiturate. Blue capsules (Bluebirds) with a strip of blue at the halfway mark on the capsule.

Anileridine – (Lerinold, Leritine). Synthetic morphinelike drug.

Atropine – Found in nightshade (belladonna) and also synthesized to treat ulcers. Large doses depress the nervous system, cause coma/death.

Benzedrine – (Bennies). Nervous system stimulant used to treat obesity, depressed persons, etc. It comes in three-sided, pink tablets with a groove in the middle (5 and 10 milligrams) and also in time-released capsules (15 milligrams).

Biphetamine – (Black Beauties). A stimulant. Sold in caps with RJS printed on them. 12½ milligrams – half black and half white. 20 milligrams – all black. Made with d-amphetamine and dl-amphetamine.

Busitol Sodium – A medium barbiturate. Flat, round green,

pink, or lavender tabs with McNeil on them.

Chloral Hydrate — The proverbial Mickey Finn. A hypnotic drug producing sleep at quantities of ½ to 1 gram.

Cyclazocine — A methadonelike synthetic narcotic used for curing narcotic addiction.

Delephine — (Methadone Hydrochloride). Morphinelike drug sold in pills and cough syrup.

Demerol — A nonaddictive, synthetic narcotic resembling morphine in effect. Often used by medical personnel instead of morphine.

Desbutal — An amphetamine and barbiturate in combination.

Desoxyn — Amphetamine stimulant. Sold in tabs and caps with a small "a" printed on them.

Dexamyl — An amphetamine/barbiturate combination. Sold in Spansules (green cap with clear green body, filled with green and white mini-tabs,) and in three-sided, green scored tablets.

Dexedrine-Amphetamine Sulfate — A powerful stimulant. Sold in liquid, caps, and tabs. Time-released caps come in 5, 10, and 15 mils and have a brown top and clear bottom. Printed SKF. Two small dots by SKF indicate 15 mils; one dot, 10 mils; no dots, 5 mils. Tabs are orange flats with a middle score and contain 5 milligrams.

Dilaudid — Synthetic derivative of morphine, with a stronger effect than morphine. Sold in pills, cough syrups, and suppositories.

Doriden — (Glutethimide). Hypnotic sedative. White, flat tablets with CIBA printed on them.

Homatropine — Synthetic derivative of atropine.

Librium — A light tranquilizer. Much less effect (i.e. high) than opiates or barbiturates. Sold in caps; 5 milligrams — green/yellow, 10 mils — brown/green. Both are inscribed with ROCHE and 25 mils — green/white.

Liertine — (Anileridein). A synthetic opiate that is less potent than morphine. Sold in white tablets. Injections can be highly dangerous.

Meperidine — A synthetic drug. While unlike morphine in chemical makeup, it strongly resembles it in bodily reactions.

Meprobamate — A light tranquilizer (sold as Miltown, Quanil, Equanil, etc.) prescribed for depressants, epileptics, etc. Habit forming to some degree.

Methadone — A synthetic opiate, which acts much like morphine in a "normal" user (relieves pain, produces euphoric effect, etc.), but in an addict, it does not produce the euphoric, smack high, but alleviates withdrawal and heroin craving.

Nalline — A derivative of morphine, which, unlike its potent cousin, produces no analgesic effects, and in fact, tends to reserve the action of the opiate group. In a normal, nondrugged soul, Nalline produces a slight feeling of relaxation and drowsiness, but in those who have used some opiate drug in the recent past, Nalline produces fairly pronounced withdrawal symptoms. Because of this side effect, it is given to parolees in California and other forward-looking states to see if they have been using a no-no.

Nembutal — A short-acting barbiturate (Yellow jackets, Nemmies). Sold in 30 milligram yellow caps with an "a" printed on them. 50 mil caps with yellow/white combination and the "a", and 100 mil caps which are all yellow with the wording ABBOTT.

Percodan — A class A narcotic used by some hardup addicts. Sold in pink scored tabs.

Pyrahexl — A THC derivative used in experimental drug withdrawal problems.

Sansert — A drug used in preventing migraine headaches, which chemically resembles LSD. Claims for heavy psychotropic properties have been made. Yellow, coated tablets (2 milligrams).

Scopolamine — A sedative and muscle relaxant derived from such organic sources as henbane and belladonna. Similar to atropine. Causes a high and hallucinations in the larger, near fatal doses. Occasionally, it is employed as a "truth serum." It appears in small quantities in over the counter drugs like Sleep-eze and Sominex, etc.

Thorazine — A tranquilizer given to patients needing major sedation. Also an LSD antagonist, i.e., reverses the effects of LSD.

Tuinal — A hypnotic sedative made from Amytal and Seconal. Sold in ½, ¾, and 3 grain caps with a blue bottom/orange top (rainbows).

Valium — Minor tranquilizer. Sold in white tabs of 2 and 5 mils. Wording — ROCHE.

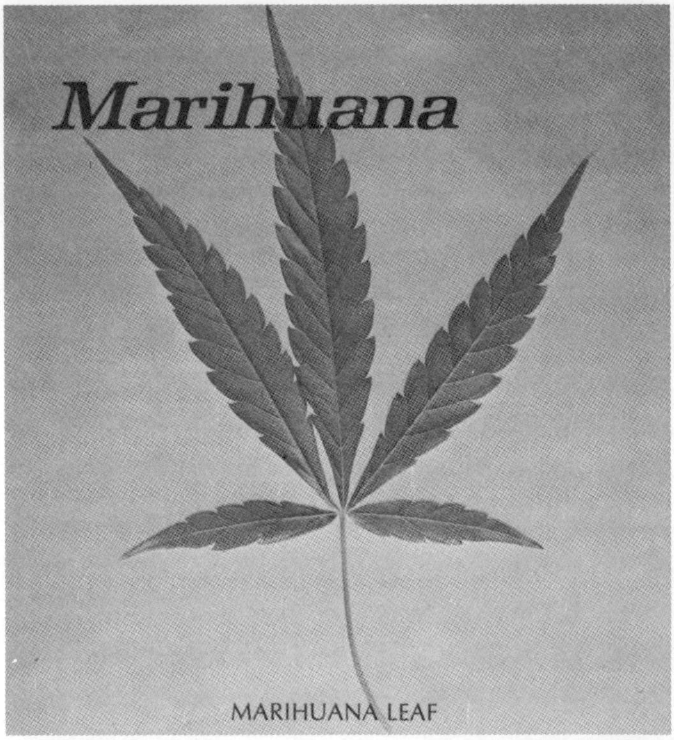

MARIHUANA LEAF

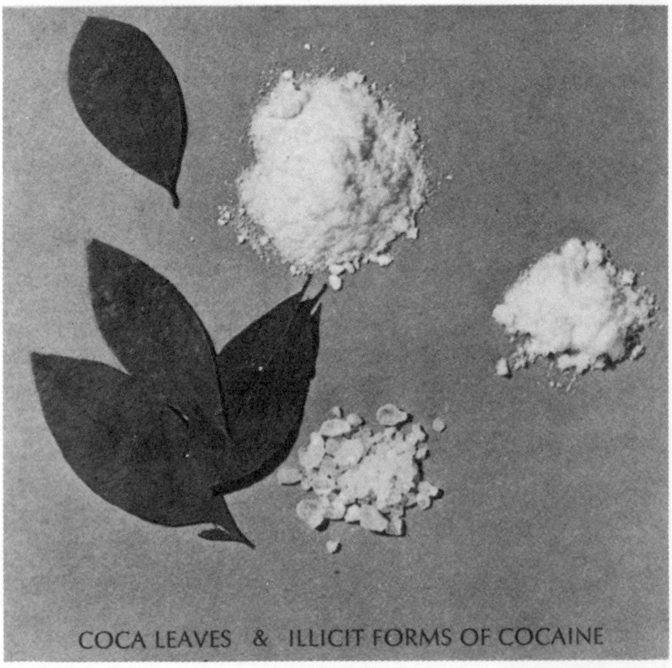

COCA LEAVES & ILLICIT FORMS OF COCAINE

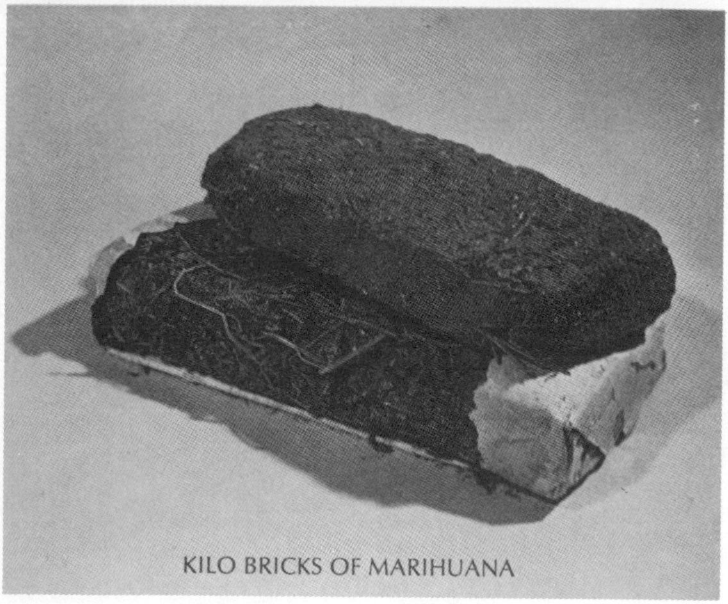

KILO BRICKS OF MARIHUANA

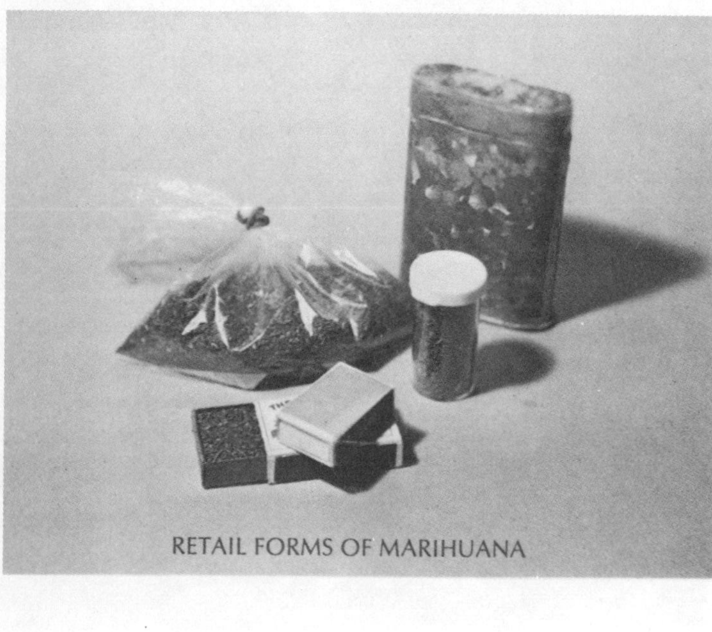

RETAIL FORMS OF MARIHUANA

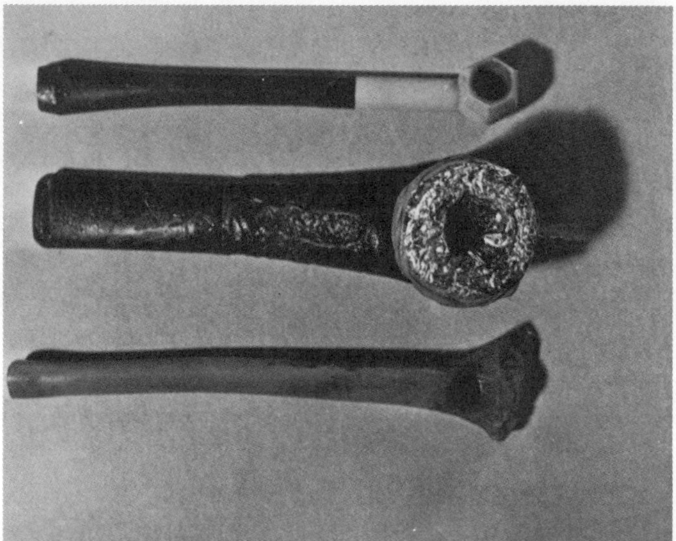

MAKESHIFT MARIHUANA PIPES

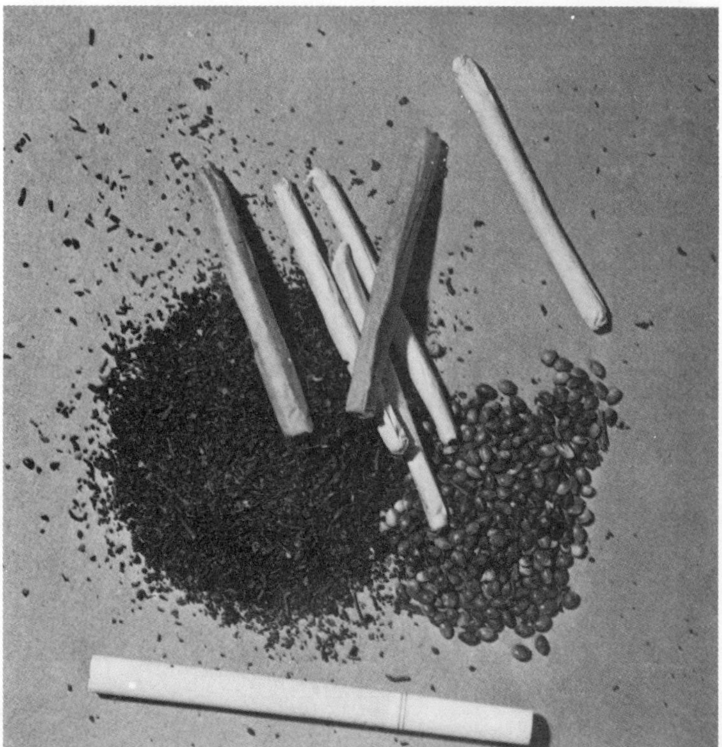

MANICURED MARIHUANA, CIGARETTES AND SEEDS

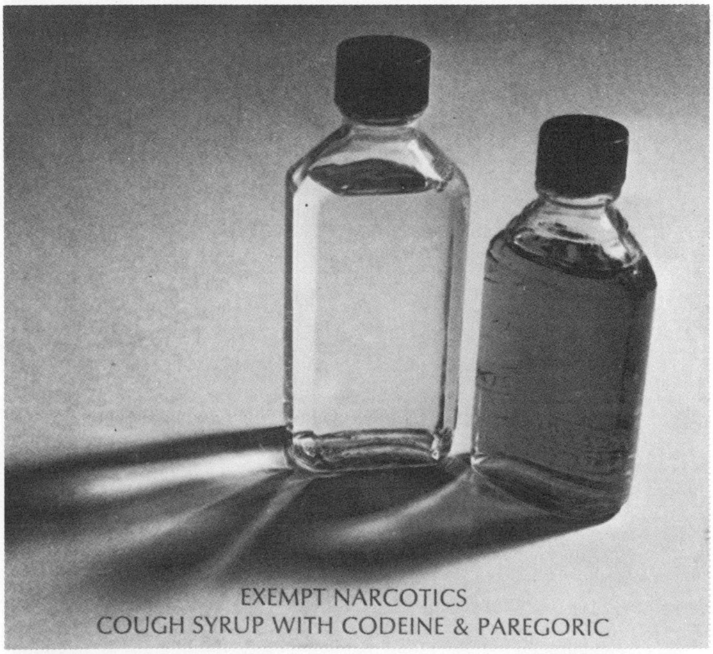

EXEMPT NARCOTICS
COUGH SYRUP WITH CODEINE & PAREGORIC

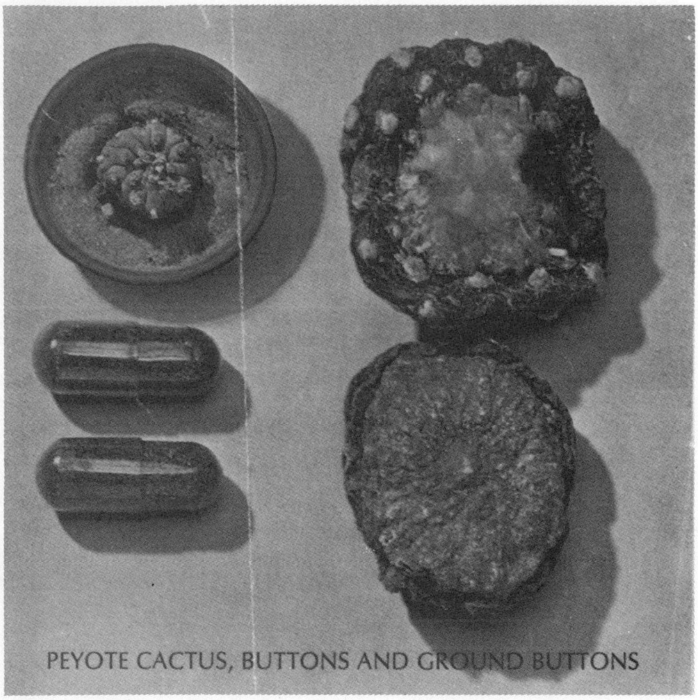

PEYOTE CACTUS, BUTTONS AND GROUND BUTTONS

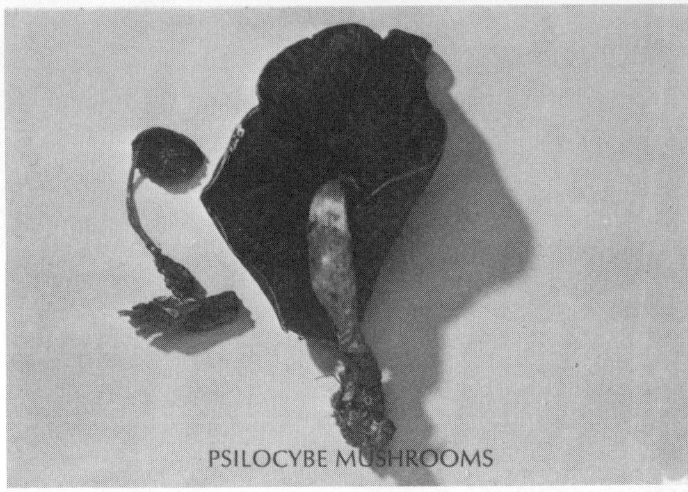

PSILOCYBE MUSHROOMS

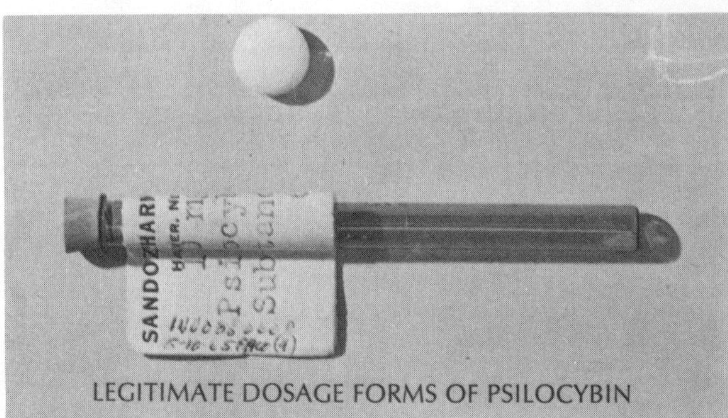

LEGITIMATE DOSAGE FORMS OF PSILOCYBIN

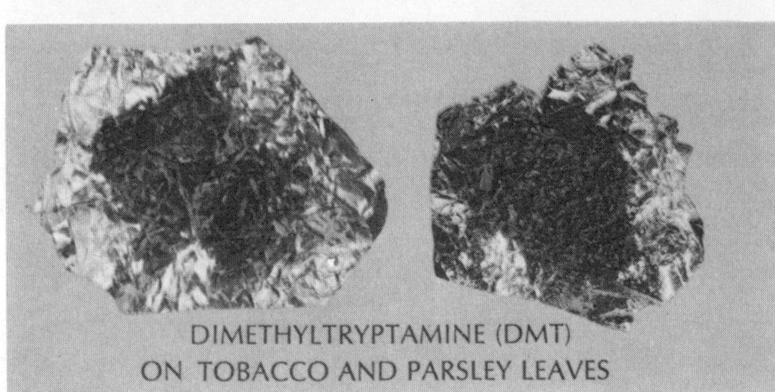

DIMETHYLTRYPTAMINE (DMT)
ON TOBACCO AND PARSLEY LEAVES

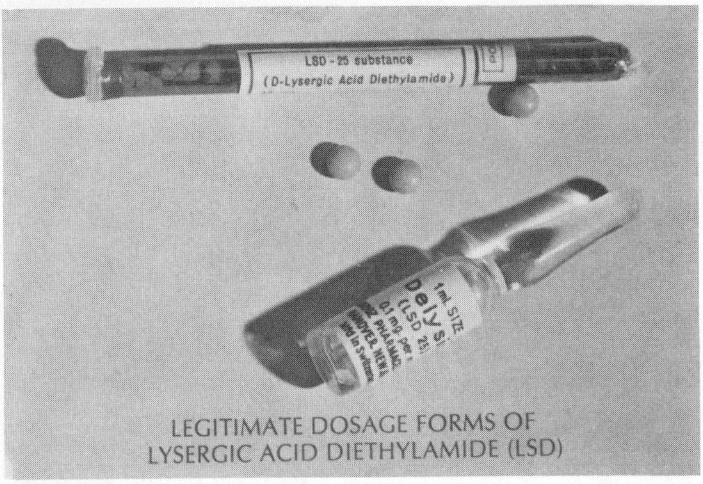

LEGITIMATE DOSAGE FORMS OF
LYSERGIC ACID DIETHYLAMIDE (LSD)

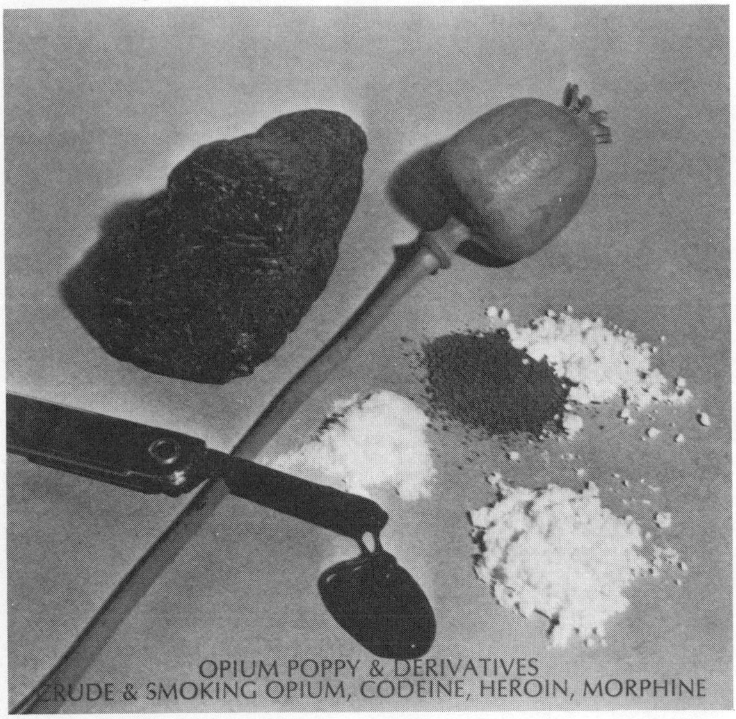

OPIUM POPPY & DERIVATIVES
CRUDE & SMOKING OPIUM, CODEINE, HEROIN, MORPHINE

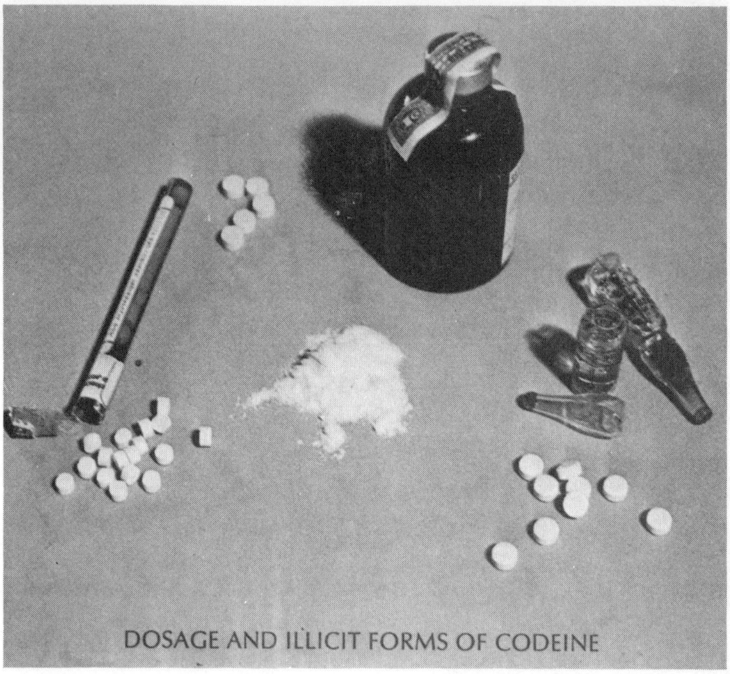

DOSAGE AND ILLICIT FORMS OF CODEINE

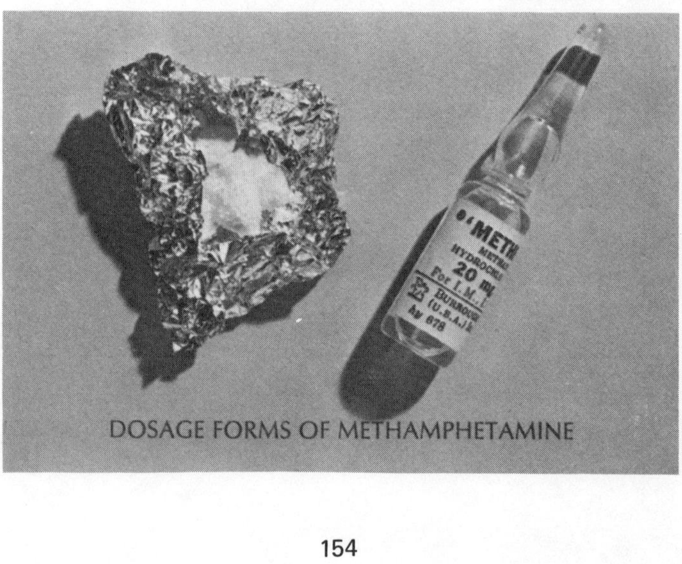

DOSAGE FORMS OF METHAMPHETAMINE

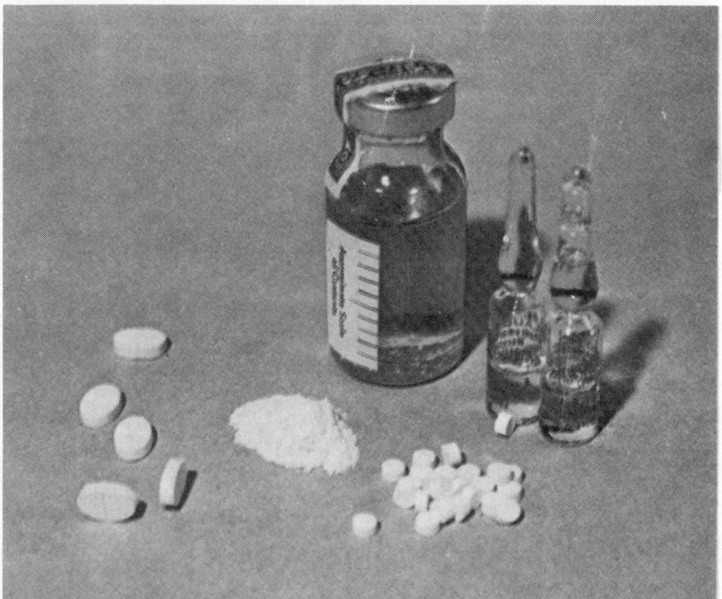

DOSAGE FORMS OF HYDROMORPHONE

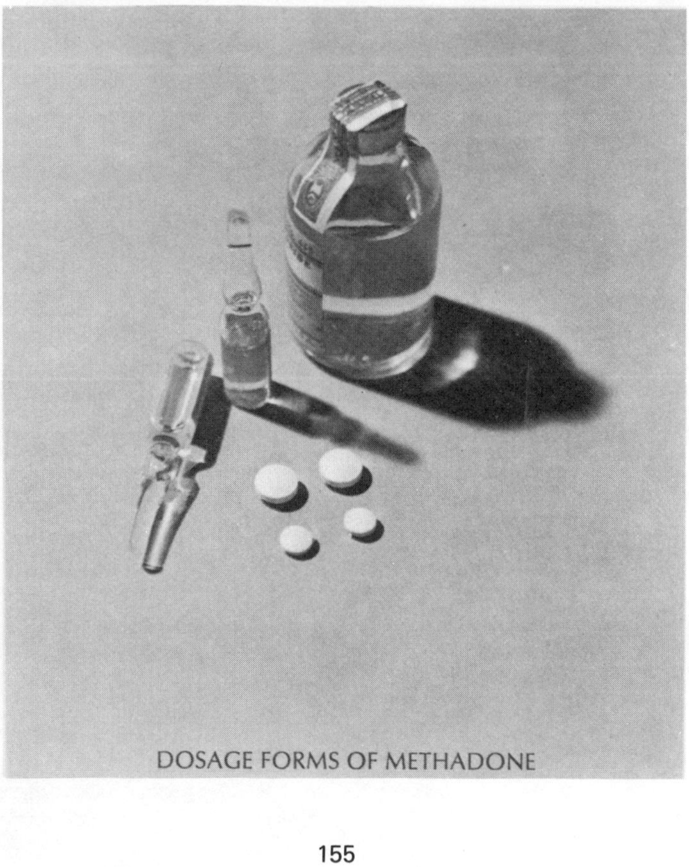

DOSAGE FORMS OF METHADONE

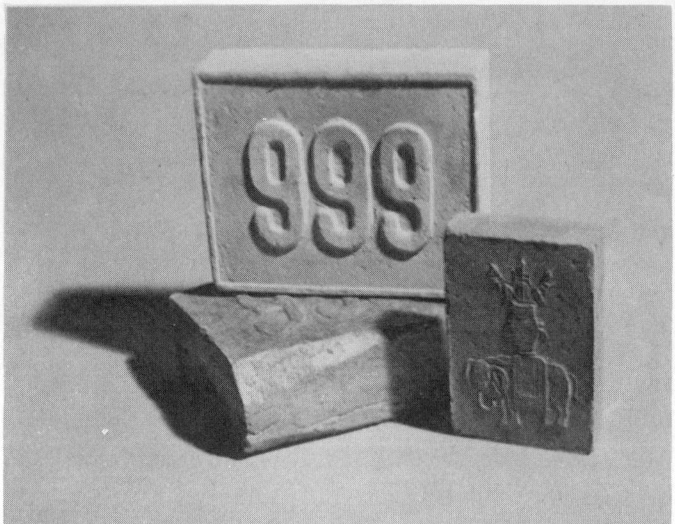

MORPHINE BASE

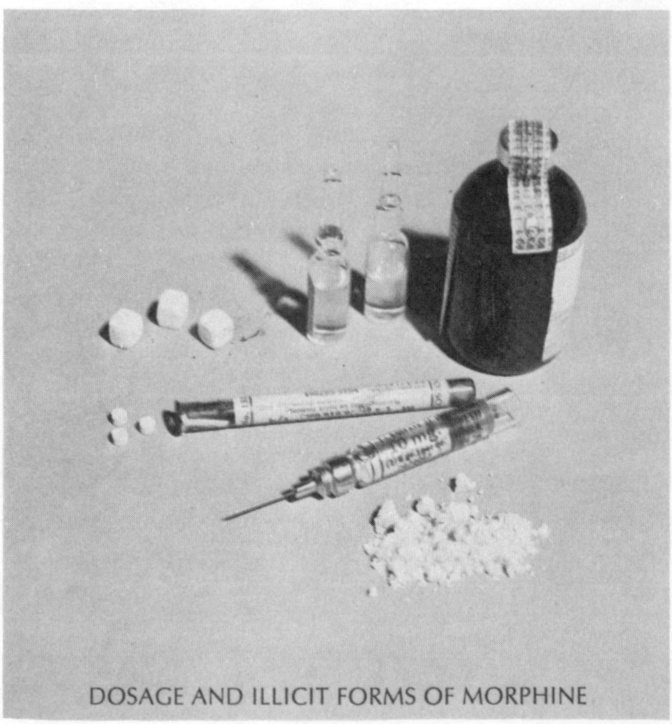

DOSAGE AND ILLICIT FORMS OF MORPHINE

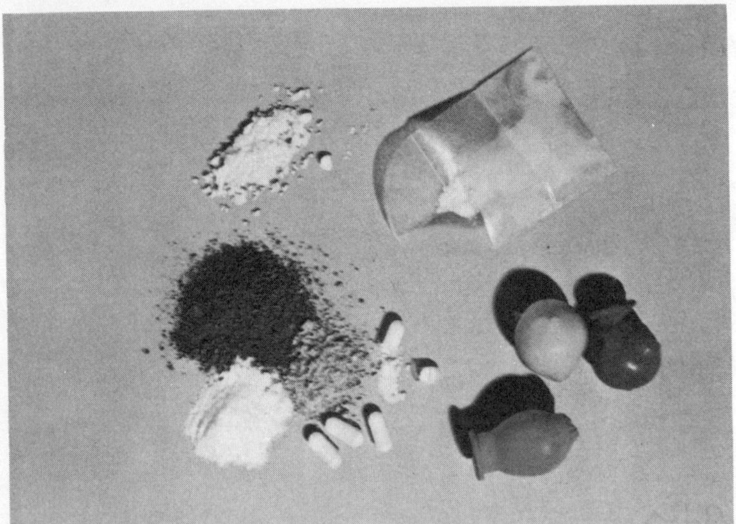

FORMS OF HEROIN

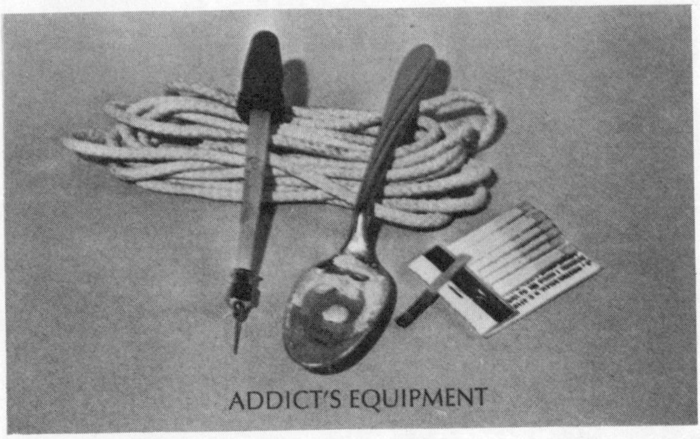

ADDICT'S EQUIPMENT

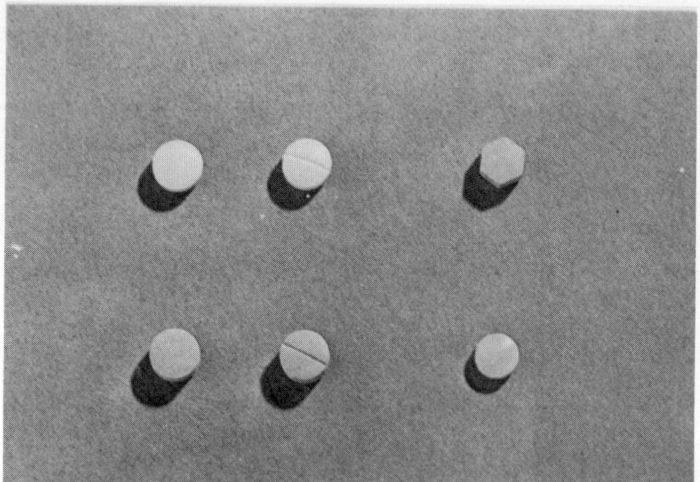

PHENOBARBITAL TABLETS

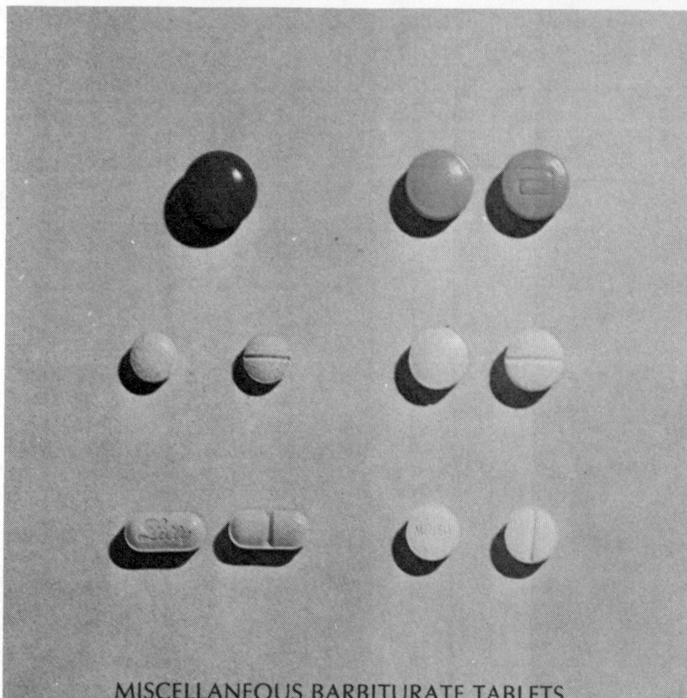

MISCELLANEOUS BARBITURATE TABLETS

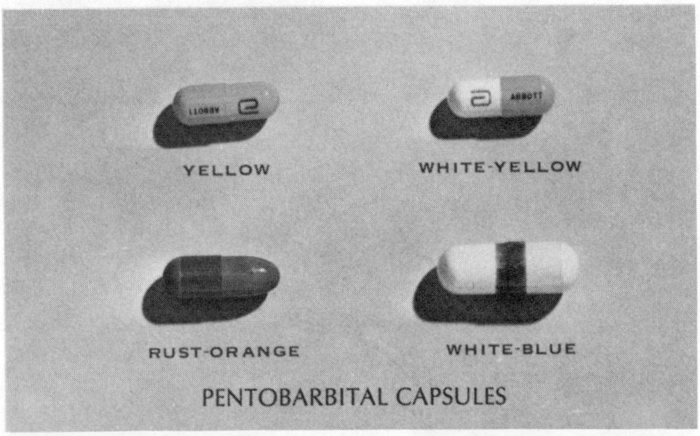

PENTOBARBITAL CAPSULES

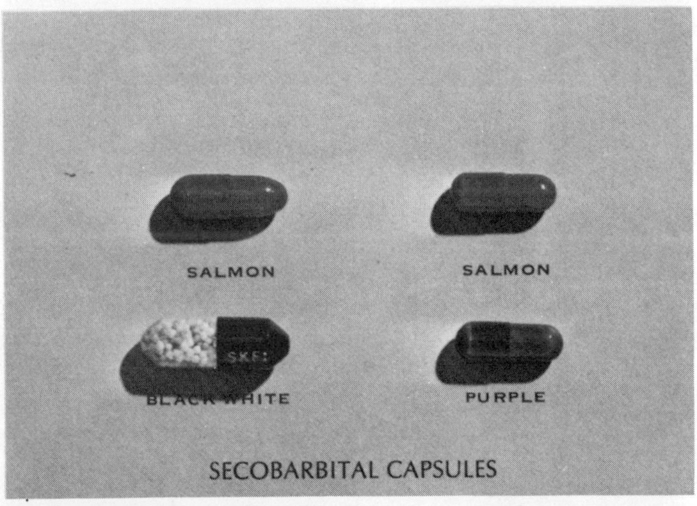

SECOBARBITAL CAPSULES

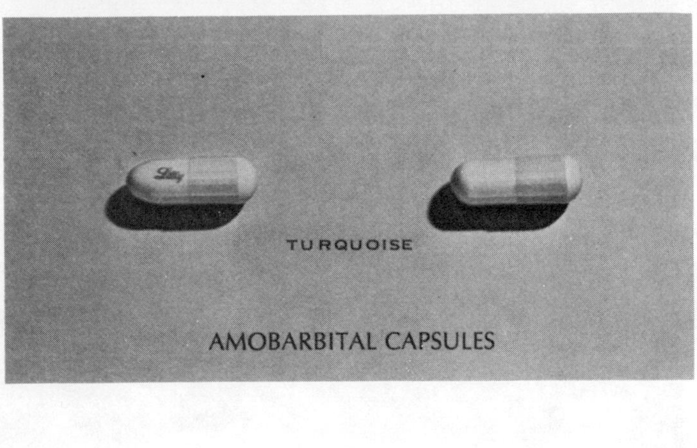

AMOBARBITAL CAPSULES

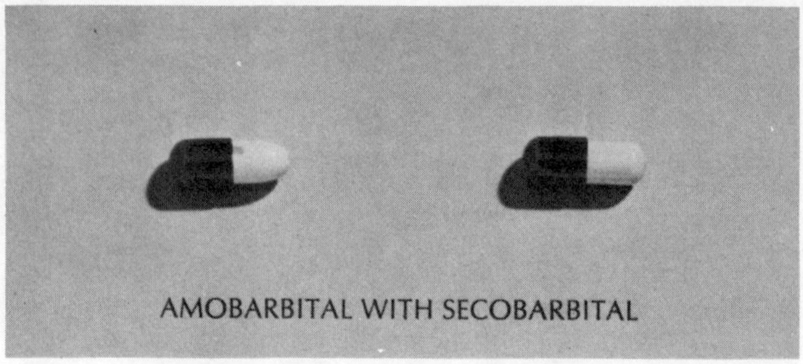

AMOBARBITAL WITH SECOBARBITAL

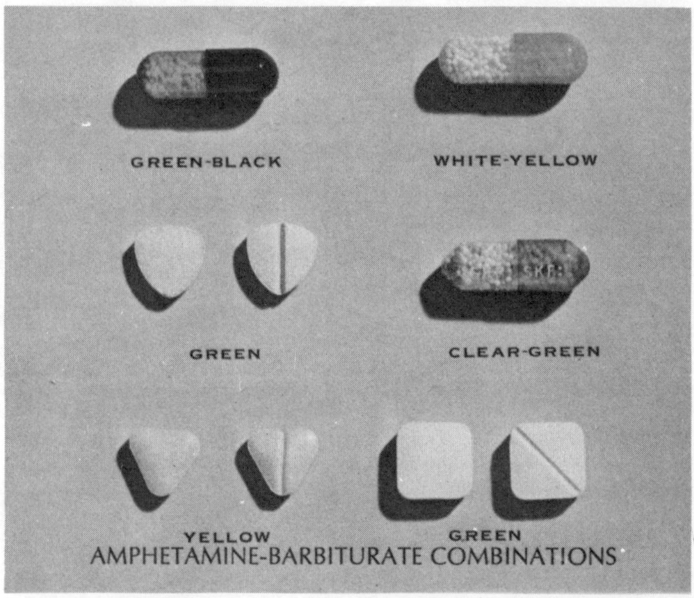

AMPHETAMINE-BARBITURATE COMBINATIONS

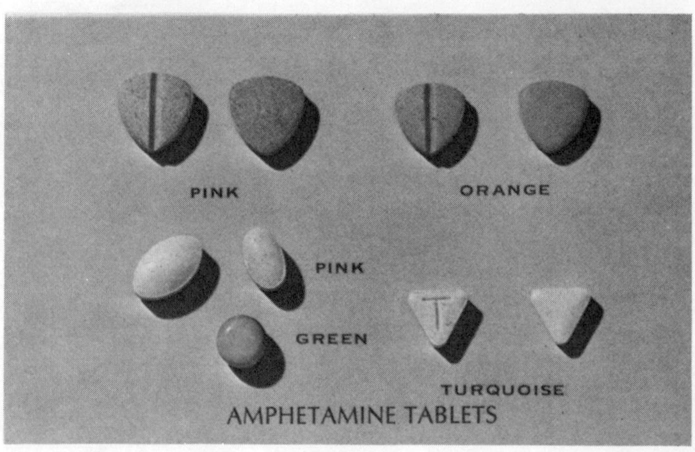

AMPHETAMINE TABLETS

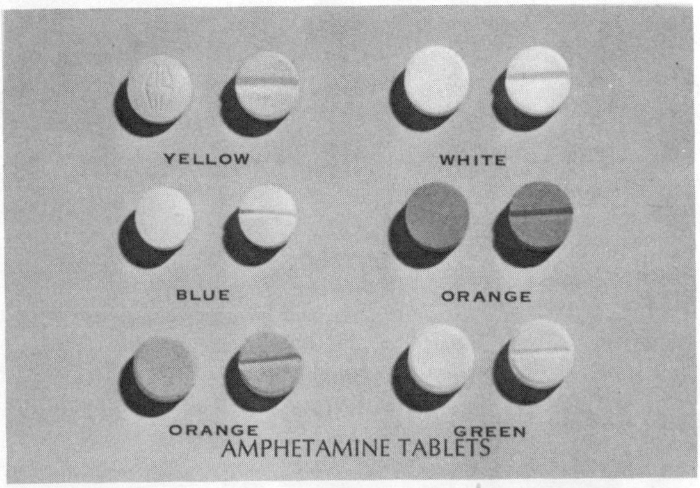

AMPHETAMINE TABLETS

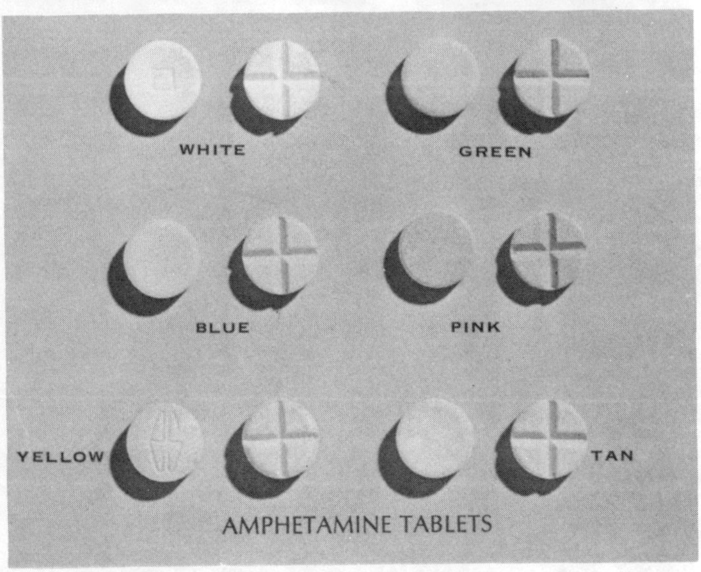

AMPHETAMINE TABLETS

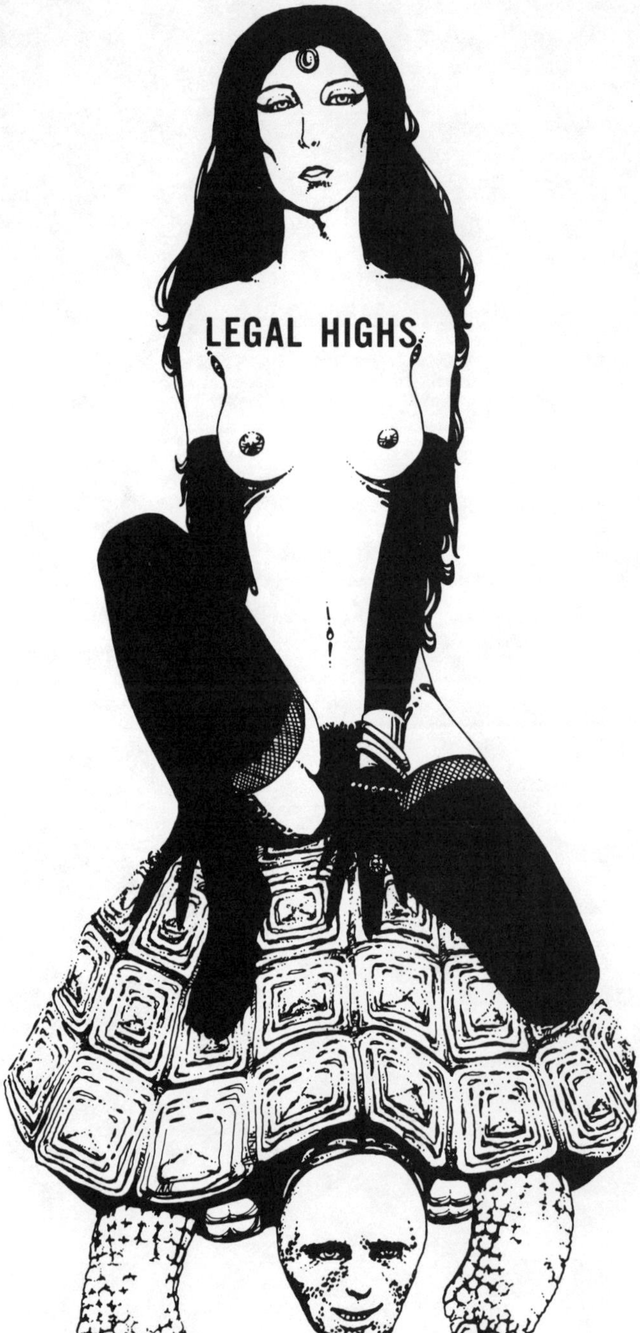
LEGAL HIGHS

LEGAL HIGHS

Many things which produce a narcotic or psychotropic reaction in the user are still legal in the United States (although this list changes almost on a monthly basis). Not all legal or cheap highs are necessarily good and not all are good for you.

Still, if you prefer to be legal whenever possible, and in most cases, organic, this could be the way to go. Most of these drugs are available with a bit of searching. However, you could still be in trouble for selling them to your friends without a license or such.

Many of these surrogate psychedelics contain an organic substitute of an outlawed drug, but they are not outlawed in their natural format.

Many legal highs are now in use in so-called "primitive" cultures around the world, and some have been used in the U.S., at one time or another. A good example of this is good old-fashioned licorice, which used to be available at every drug counter, and was often prescribed for coughs and sore throats and is a mild opiate.

NEVER TAKE ANY DRUG OR PLANT IN ANY MANNER OTHER THAN FOR WHICH IT IS INTENDED OR ADVISED. Foolish as it seems, people have been hospitalized, and in at least one case, have died from shooting (injecting) the extract of boiled marijuana.

Many legal highs fall into the category of MOA (monoamine oxidase) inhibitors. This is a group of amphetamine-related drugs which act as central nervous system stimulants and mood uppers.

Some MOA inhibitors are being prescribed in psychotic disorder treatments. The popular drugs in the class are Marplan, Niamid, Parnate, and Eutonyl.

MOA inhibitors interfere with the normal enzymes (monoamine oxidase) which works to neutralize the natural bodily stimulants (cathecholamines) after they have stimulated a neuron. This prolongs the nerve stimulation to unnatural levels. They can also mess up the amine levels which may take a few days or even weeks to return to normal.

All this means: if you are going to experiment with MOA inhibitors, NEVER, NEVER mix them with other drugs (including prescription drugs such as insulin): NEVER use any other drug within a few days after or before tripping with MOA drugs; and for some unexplained reason, NEVER eat cheese and go easy on milk products when using these drugs.

Needless to say, NEVER drink alcohol with any MOA drug.

BETEL NUTS

Used by millions of poeple in the Asiatic countries, the betel nut is actually the seed of a large tree. The nut is combined with other spices (sometimes nutmeg) and sucked in the mouth for hours, much as Americans with an oral fetish satisfy themselves with gum.

The betel is a nervous system stimulant, although prolonged use stains the lips and teeth a bright red, and it is said to weaken one sexually after some time.

BROOM

Several types of broom (a member of the bean family found in the U.S.) can be aged for a couple of weeks, dried, and smoked. The smoking is done much as with grass, and a mild relaxing high with mescaline like color intensification is experienced.

BROOM MUST NEVER BE EATEN – JUST SMOKED.

CALIFORNIA POPPY

Hurrah for California! They have not only popularized but immortalized a narcotic by making the state flower none other then the California Poppy.

The flower's leaves are dried and smoked, and the stems are sometimes boiled into a tea. The plant contains several opiates or opiate like substances (protopine, sanguinarine, etc.), but is not habit forming. It is only a mild intoxicant, but the effects could probably be increased through some sort of process similar to making hash oil.

CANARY WEED

The blossoms, leaves, and maybe beans, of the plant Genista canariensis give a mild high when smoked. Available in nurseries in the U.S.

CLUB MOSS

Club moss, Lycopdium gnidiodes is reported to give a marijuana like high when smoked. The plant's cousins are found in the U.S. and may be looked up in a botany text.

COLEUS

A plant of the mint family, Coleus is grown in the U.S. and employed by hard-up Indians as a replacement for psychedelic mushrooms. It is not as potent but of definite psychotic nature.

Coleus blumei and Coleus pumilius are both employed for extracurricular activities. C. blumei is the commoner variety, being a perennial herb reaching a height of three feet, while C. pumilius sort of just lies there or falls over the pot edges.

Both types do best with plenty of water and a loose, rich soil. The seeds should be started indoors in shallow starting boxes (bottom heat helps) and transplanted after all frost danger is past.

They both do well from cuttings which have been soaked in water to start the roots. An organic fertilizer with a high nitrogen content benefits Coleus.

The leaves and flowers are eaten to produce the psychotropic effects. The leaves seem to work only fresh, not when dried and should be frozen for extended storage. Quite a few leaves (50 or so) are required for at rip.

DAMIANA

A shrub which is found in California, Texas, and other states with a similar climate, which may be boiled for tea or the leaves smoked (after drying) to give a slight grass like high, although some say a prolonged use may damage the liver.

DONANA

A small cactus found in Texas which contains a peyotelike combination of alkaloids. About ten small cacti are eaten on an empty stomach, after removing the spines.

HARMALINE

Occurring in several plants, Harmaline is used by several tribes and races of our South American cousins. Most of these compounds need about 200 mg (orally) to be psychotropically active.

HAWAIIAN BABY WOOD ROSE SEEDS

A popular drug with the "in" crowd for some time. HBWR seeds are most often ordered direct from a Hawaiian nursery. Some have gotten hip and refuse to sell, while others are only too happy to ship to the mainland at a higher price than they can get in Hawaii. This one is a natural for some sort of government hassling.

The active ingredients include D-lysergic acid amides and other related compounds.

The usual dose is about four - eight seeds which are removed from their seed pods and the outer white layer scraped away. The seeds are now eaten whole or ground and soaked as with morning glory seeds.

The seeds produce an acid like high which lasts for about five - six hours.

One person we know tried to order from a number of Hawaiian suppliers by telephone (with a fake credit card number, of course) and received a variety of responses from people simply hanging up to "sorry, all out." Finally, one supplier said, "Gee, I am all sold out to the mainland again this season. Man, there must be one heck of a lot of Wood Rose Plants growing in California."

HEIMA

Grows in South America and one or two species in Texas. Reported to be psychedelic but no facts are known.

HOPS

A fairly close relative of marijuana, hops will give a slight high if dried and smoked. The problem here is that a popular drug book showed how to graft hops and grass together to produce a non-marijuana appearing hybrid which still packed the ol' wallop, and the government has asked suppliers not to sell the general public any seeds or plants.

KAVA KAVÁ

Piper methysticum and Pierr plantagiveum are chewed by various Mexican and hip Caribbeans to give a slight grass like, relaxed high. Needs at least three grams to be felt.

MEXICAN MINT

Mexican Mint (Salvia divinorum) can be chewed for its hallucinogenic agents. Its American cousins (purple sage, etc.) don't seem to contain the active ingredients.

Can be purchased in certain nurseries in the US. The Mexicans chew about 50 - 60 leaves and cross their fingers.

MIMOSA

The roots of the plants in the Mimosa genus are supposed to contain an organic form of DMT.

MORNING GLORY

One of the original of the organic highs, several varieties, including: Heavenly Blue, Pearly Gates, Wedding Bells, etc. may be utilized.

The active parts include amides of lysergic acid, chanoclavine, and clymoclavine, all of which are found in the natural ergot which contains modern LSD.

As might be expected, the morning glory trip is very much like a LSD jaunt. The seeds are about one-tenth as potent as LSD ergot and it takes about five - ten grams for an average trip.

Some seeds are covered with methyl mercury to prevent spoilage or with vomit inducers to discourage psychotropic uses. If the treated seeds are planted, the next generation will be clean. It is possible to buy "organic" untreated seeds.

A little protection can be gotten by grinding the seeds into a powder and then soaking in cold water for an hour or so. The water is stained and drunk.

NO_2

Laughing gas, or nitrous oxide, is a pleasant, fairly safe little "trip." Mild euphoric and dreamy state. More than a few inhalations will produce a dizziness-sleep state.

Do not breathe directly from the tank (let it warm up in a balloon or bag first) and if using a mask, do not fit tightly over the face. Should have at least 20 per cent O_2 or air in the gas.

NUTMEG

Nutmeg has been a popular cheap high in prisons for a number of years, but its unpleasant side effects make the trip doubtful for any free person. It contains an MDA-like substance which imparts a dreamy mescaline like state for a number of hours.

In order to get off, one must consume about 15 - 20 grams of nutmeg. It can also be purchased in an oil form which is more concentrated, but which is all but unpalatable.

RAT ROOT

Acorus calamus (also called flag) grows in much of the world and is chewed by Canadian Indians for fun and excitement in, one must presume, Saturday night rituals.

The active ingredient seems to be a hallucinogenic amphetamine.

SAN PEDRO CACTUS

Native to Peru, the San Pedro cactus can be purchased in the States with little problem. About six - eight inches of the "stem" is peeled and eaten, preferably over a period of time.

Contains mescaline among other things.

SWEET FLAG

The roots of the Sweet Flag (found in the U.S.) contain a drug known as Asarone, which can also be purchased alone. It is related to TMA, or turns into a TMA-related drug in the digestive system and is quite a bit more potent than mescaline.

A normal dose is about 100-200 mg taken on an empty stomach, but this can vary widely with the user.

WORMWOOD

A narcotic herb common in the U.S. of A. The good parts are extracted by mixing with some alcohol (usually Pernod) and the liquid consumed. This may be habit forming.

YOHIMBE

An African tree which can be purchased in the U.S. About five - ten teaspoons of the inner bark is boiled for fifteen minutes in a a pint of water and then 500 mg of vitamin C is added, and the mixture is sipped as one would a fine tea.

A light high with perceptual changes and an aphrodisiac like condition is produced.

NON-ORGANIC

ALPHA CHOLRALOSE

Alpha cholralose is produced by reacting chloral with glucose under heat and is similar to PCP in reaction but with minimal side effects.

5-FLOURO-A-METHLYTRYPTAMINE

Synthetic, but legal. If about 25 mg is consumed a mescaline like high is experienced.

5-MeO-DMT

This is another example of an organic, legal drug with an obvious illegal counterpart. 5-Me-O-DMT is found in the bark of several South American plants which are still (how long, how long?) legal in the U.S.

Several underground chemists have extracted 5-Me-O and are packing it in the best Madison Avenue style and selling it quite openly.

A small (3-5 mg) dose taken on an empty stomach will produce an LSD-like high for about a half hour. It is usually mixed with some inert substance and smoked or can be sniffed.

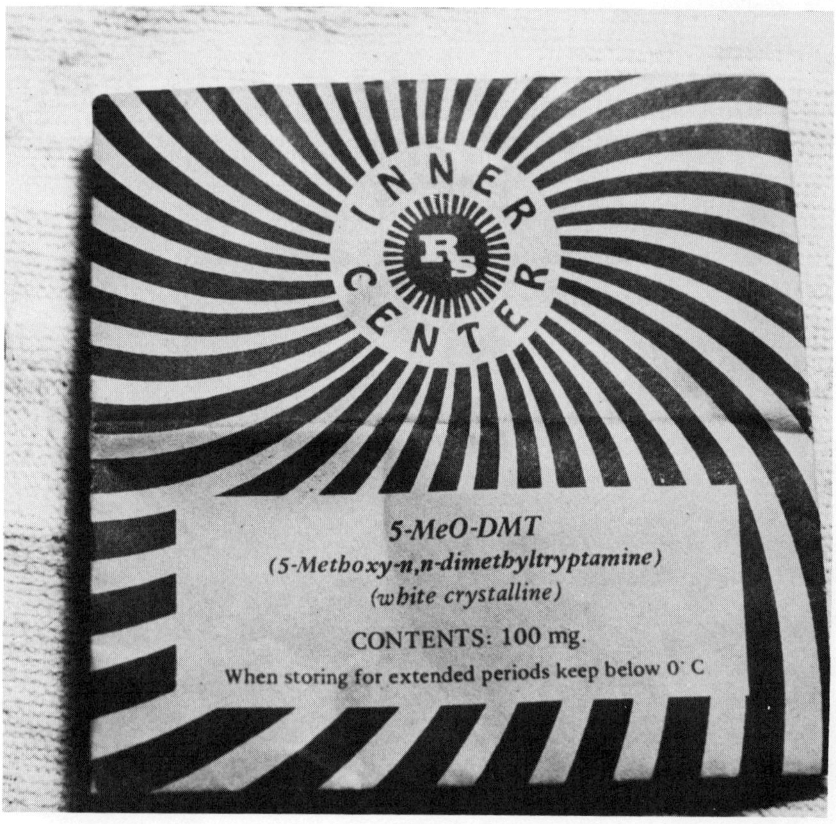

BADDIES

There are quite a number of organic highs with side effects bordering on disaster which should be avoided.

BANANA

Smoking bananas helps no one except the United Fruit Company.

BELLADONNA

Either in flower form (nightshade) or in commercial preparations such as Asthmador, Belladonna is a no-no.

It was used by witches in times past to convince the user he/she/it was flying and seeing demons. This thought alone should give one some pause before using.

It is a very toxic substance, and the difference between a deadly dose and a trip is very narrow. Users often hallucinate bugs, crabs, snakes, monsters, germs, and so on. Most trips are quite unpleasant somewhere along the way.

DILL AND PARSLEY

Both the oil of dill and parsley cause a slight high, but both are harmful to the digestive system.

JIMSON WEED

Datura stramonium, or Jimson weed has gained a sudden popularity with the publishing of Carlos Castenada books describing the use of Jimson weed for religious truisms.

Native users make a tea of the roots or leaves, or even smoke the leaves. U.S. freaks seem more inclined to go right to the source, so to speak, and eat the plant's fruit.

Jimson grows to an average height of two-three feet and is a dusty green with yellow or purple blossoms. It contains a hyoscyamine and scopolamine and even a bit of atropine.

The fruit resembles the fruit of the chestnut with an outer covering of prickly hairs. It can grow to an inch or two, and upon maturity is a dark green color. An average fruit contains about 100 seeds.

Upon ingestion, the atropine causes fever rushes and hallucinations. Overindulgence can throw the user into a coma.

A typical trip is a relaxed feeling with a difficulty in focusing the eyes. Visual hallucinations are common and often the user is unable to recall his actions after the drug has worn off.

Side effects include vomiting, headache, and loss of muscular coordination. The trip can vary from very pleasant to downright horrible with an alarming frequency.

It is often sold as WOLFBANE, it is needless to say, not.

JUNIPER

It is sometimes used by Indians to induce a dizzy, hypnotic trance state. The victim inhales the smoke and often feels he is near death or God. He is usually correct.

THORN APPLE

Thorn Apple in one form or another is drunk or eaten by the locals in India and causes blacking out, coupled with a form of insanity which can be either temporary or permanent, and occasionally, ends in death.

SNIFFING

You are what you inhale.

There are many substances which are highly toxic to the body (such as strychnine and other poisons) which produce a highly psychedelic state prior to the time the death level is reached (one can only presume they also do this in death levels).

Some, such as petroleum distillates, glue, acetone, hydrocarbons, etc., produce oxygen starvation to the brain cells and replace the O_2

with toxic counterparts. This produces a poisoned state in which the user staggers about, goes into uncontrollable fits of laughter, and suffers manic depression.

It also has the effect of destroying brain tissue each and every time it is used. When someone staggers around sniffing glue from the brown paper bag, he is not high, just too fucking STUPID to know his brain is being poisoned. Each time one indulges, more and more cells go, and the user gets stupider and stupider.

A common sight in prison is the long-timer who uses cleaning fluid from the laundry to keep happy every night. The guards are happy because the nut is in a stupor much of the time, and the other inmates soon learn to avoid the sniffer like the plague as he begins slurring words and going into depression fits.

GASOLINE, PAINT THINNER, ETC.

The hydrocarbons in these products cause effects similar to intoxication as well as buzzing in the ears and weird noises. Heavy doses can cause coma states, seizures, and brain damage.

GLUE

Good ol' airplane glue. This nice stuff swells membranes, causes anemia, damages the brain and kidneys, and stops the bones from making blood.

The body's attempts to reject the poison is what makes you feel stoned. Wisely, most manufacturers today are adding oil of mustard or other vomit inducers to glues.

Cheap highs are not worth it. Save up and buy a lid.

PAM, PAINT, HAIR SPRAYS

The "stone" in these products is not in the ingredients but rather in the propellants, such as Freon. The propellant produces a short "rush" when ingested, but it is impossible to separate the propellant from the gunk and so your lungs get a good dose of hair spray, vegetable oil, etc.

Freon also has the nice effect of freezing living tissue. Several people have died from this little unpleasantry, usually from inhaling cocktail glass chillers. IF YOU JUST GOTTA USE FREON, at least let it go into a balloon and warm up for a half hour or so. . .

CHURCH OF THE TREE OF LIFE
451 Columbus Avenue
San Francisco, California 94133

Supporting members ($10 or more per year) get a membership card, book of teachings, certificate, the First Book of Sacraments, supplements to the Book, a quarterly newsletter and a free question-answering service, catalogs of reliable suppliers of legal drugs, recommended reading lists, information releases, etc.

Donating members ($5 or more per year) get card, certificate, newsletter, book of teachings, info releases, catalogs, etc.

Assisting members (less than $5 but more than $1) get card, book of teachings, current issue of newsletter, some current info releases.

Gratis members ($1 or less) regarded as members but receive no free materials.

The Church of the Tree of Life is a nondogmatic, nonprofit religious organization which has been legally incorporated in the State of California since November 3, 1971. During our first year, without the aid of any contrived publicity, we have gained more than 1,500 members throughout the USA, and we continue to add at least 100 new members each month. We also have some members in other countries.

We do not preach about God, afterlife, or sin and virtue. We have no firsthand knowledge on these subjects and therefore have no business imposing our personal feelings or beliefs upon our members. What you believe is your own business. The only essential belief of our Church is that the human being is sovereign of his/her own mind and body and must have the right to do with himself/herself or with any consenting adults whatever he/she pleases, as long as his/her actions do not violate the rights of others.

SACRAMENTS

Although we do not press the point as religious dogma, most of us tend to feel that all substances in the universe are nature's gifts to us and that we may select any of these to fulfill our tastes and requirements. We believe in the right of the individual to make all decisions regarding his private behavior and to use whatever substances he wishes as medicines, nutriments, mind alterants, etc. We cannot officially embrace as sacraments illegal substances such as marijuana and LSD. Other churches which attempted to do this have failed. What we can do and have done is to declare as sacraments all substances that are presently legal. You may recall that during liquor prohibition churches and synagogues were allowed to continue to use sacramental wine. Members of the Native American Church (mostly Indians) are permitted to use peyote in their services because it had been their sacrament before laws were passed against it. Many of our sacraments, such as yohimbe, kava kava, Hawaiian wood rose, morning glory, San Pedro and Donana cacti, and even vitamins (see new FDA ruling) are in danger of legislative control and prohibition. It was not our original intention to conspire to inhibit legislation, but if any of our sacraments are made illegal in the future, the government cannot deny their use to church members without directly and clearly violating our constitutional guarantee of religious freedom.

Since freedom without knowledge and wisdom leads to chaos, we recognize our responsibility to impart to our members information and advice on the proper use of these sacraments. We do this through our various publications including BARK LEAF (quarterly bulletin), books such as THE FIRST BOOK OF SACRAMENTS, supplementary reports, annotated bibliographies of recommended reading, lists of reliable suppliers of sacraments, and a Xeroxed information research service. As we grow, we create new publications. We are now developing a library and reading room for our members.

MEMBERSHIP

You may be a member of any other church and still be a member of the Church of the Tree of Life. You need not partake of any of the Church's sacraments as long as you believe in the right of the individual to make his own choices regarding the use of sacraments and other acts of private behavior.

WOODROSE/LSD EXTRACTION

Hawaiian Baby and Regular Wood Rose seeds contain a fairly large amount (relatively speaking) of organic LSD derivatives (about 3 mg of alkaloids per gram of seeds). This active derivative can be extracted and eaten or extracted and turned into real LSD.

Grind up the seeds into a fine powder and cover with 100 ml petroleum ether to each 100 gr seeds and let soak for two days. Filter the residue and throw away the ether. Let the seeds dry and add 100 ml emthanol and resoak for two days. Filter, repeat the process with another 100 ml methanol, and evaporate the two methanol extracts in a vacuum.

The remaining yellow oil contains the LSD derivatives. This oil can be chromatographically purified by a fairly complicated process which we won't go into here.

MESCALINE EXTRACTION FROM CACTI

This method will work on any of the mescaline-producing cactus found in the U.S. or Mexico. Dry the tops of the cactus and grind them up. Add 50 gr of this ground mixture to 250 ml of methanol and let it soak for 12 hours. Filter and add 100 ml 1N HCL to the damp mess and let sit for about two hours. At the same time, you should evaporate the methanol in a vacuum.

Now filter the HCL solution until clear and add to the residue obtained from the drying of the methanol. Make neutral PH (7) by adding 2N KOH and add 100 ml $CHCL_3$. Mix in a separatory funnel and separate the bottom layer. Add 40 ml water to this and separate in the funnel again. Dry and evaporate in a vacuum the remaining $CHCL_3$ to get the goodies.

GROWING YOUR OWN

It is possible to grow a number of legal (and, of course, not so legal) psychotropic plants within your own little confines. The advantages to this system are numerous: you get to experiment and exercise your own quality control, it gives you a chance to become involved with plants, and lastly, but surely not leastly, it's cheap.

GENERAL

Always endeavor to use seeds or cuttings that appear fresh and hearty. Avoid seeds which have sat for over one year or appear dried and shriveled. Some seeds will start better if soaked in water until they are swollen up (not longer than one day). Occasionally (such as with large WoodRose seeds) with a hard outer shell may have to be nicked sligthly with a sharp knife prior to soaking.

SPROUTING: Seeds can be sprouted in any number of mediums including peat moss or numerous commercial sprouting preparations. Sprouting is best accomplished in a slated sprouting box or in cut-down paper cups with a hole in the bottom. Place the seeds in a couple of times their own thickness of sprouting medium or dirt unless otherwise noted.

Bottom heating may encourage sprouting. This can be accomplished with the help of a small light bulb placed in such a way that the heat warms the bottom of the sprouting box. Pilot lights are also employed for this purpose BUT be sure your heat is low enough so not to cook the seeds, just warm them.

The plants should be transplanted to their permanent homes after the second set of leaves has opened. This should be done on a cool, cloudy day, or just after sunset. For indoor transplants utilize a green safelight. (See the mairjuana chapter for specific growth and transplanting instructions.)

Plants should be grown in loose, rich soil. Humus can be added as well as a light mixture of organic fertilizer (again, see the section on growing marijuana) and worms.

If you are growing indoors, it is wise to start with sterilized, nursery-bought soil.

SPECIFICS

Morning Glory: Morning Glories are a good starting point for those of us with purple thumbs – they grow with little help from man or beast. If you are interested in the more-than-aesthetic value, Morning Glories, you will want to purchase only: Heavenly Blue, Pearly Gates, Flying Saucers, Wedding Bells, Summer Skies, Blue Star and Badoh Negro. Avoid the other varieties as they are non-psychotropic.

The commercial seeds may be treated with chemicals to induce sickness if you attempt to eat them, but any succeeding generations will be adulterant free.

Morning Glory seeds will definitely benefit from the soaking program detailed earlier. Plant-soaked seeds under about ½" of good soil and about 6 - 7" apart. Provide some sort of support (fences, trellis, etc.) for the vines.

It is possible to assure yourself of maximum alkaloid content by influencing a couple of factors in the plant's environment: soil should be adjusted to a Ph of 6.5 and should contain quite a bit of phosphate and not much potassium (use a soil-testing kit). Adjust the values with sodium nitrate and sodium hydrophosphate.

Another possibility is to experiment with the various growth influencers as shown in the marijuana section of this book.

Remember, if you are going to use MG plants for ingestion purposes, you can get more by utilizing the whole plant instead of just the seeds. Although the seeds contain the highest amount of active goodies on a per weight basis, the other portions of the plant also contain the active alkaloids and can be extracted with methods detailed under organic chemistry.

WOOD ROSE

Both the Hawaiian Baby and Large Wood Rose plants contain an LSD alkaloid, but the baby variety seems to contain about two-three times as much as its larger cousin.

Wood Rose seeds come in a pod of four large seeds and should be nicked and soaked before planting. During the first year of growth the plant may be kept in a large pot inside your abode, but during the second year it should be moved outside to enter its vine stage, at which time it should produce flowers and seeds.

The BWR is a tropical plant and does not flourish in cold climates. If you live in an area which gets harsh winters, take the plant inside and store until spring.

CACTUS

The various types of psychedelic cacti can be grown outdoors in the West or South and indoors in the rest of the country. The cacti prefers a fairly sandy soil and are best grown (if indoors) in clay pots.

San Pedro is the most common type of psychotropic cactus, but Donana, Trichocereus, and Trichocereus macrogonus are also grown for their inner joys.

Some cacti have very small, fine seeds (such as peyote) which should be started on a bed of sand and leaf mold. The fine seeds should be scattered on top of the soil mixture and covered with a thin layer of same. Moisture is best obtained by allowing the soil to soak up small amounts.

San Pedro can be grown from seeds, but, like most cacti, this is a long, drawn-out process. A better solution is to begin with cuttings from a healthy plant. Allow the cuttings to dry for a couple of days, or until the cut surface area dries to a cork-like hardness.

The cuttings should be treated with a commercial root starter (purchased at your friendly local nursery) and placed in sterilized soil mixture containing sand, loam, and leaf mold. Water lightly or allow to soak up necessary moisture.

When you decide to harvest your crop, be sure and leave at least the root system and some of the plant so it can regrow.

Some people ascertain that additions of gypsum and superphosphate will promote flowering and thereby, seeds.

MUSHROOMS

The various types of happy mushrooms can be cultivated by the determined amateur, but the processes are quite involved and will not be detailed here. If you are interested, I would advise you to order one or more of the appropriate books from the further reading list in the back of this book.

COLEUS

A plant of the mint family, Coleus is grown in the U.S. and employed by hard-up Indians as a replacement for psychedelic mushrooms. It is not as potent but of definite psychotic nature.

Coleus blumei and Coleus pumilis are both employed for extra-curricular activities. C. blumei is the commoner variety, being a perennial herb reaching a height of three feet, while C. pumilis sort of just lies there or falls over the pot edges.

Both types do best with plenty of water and a loose, rich soil. The seeds should be started indoors in shallow starting boxes (bottom heat helps) and transplanted after all frost danger is past.

They both do well from cuttings which have been soaked in water to start the roots. An organic fertilizer with a high nitrogen content benefits Coleus.

The leaves and flowers are eaten to produce the psychotropic effects. The leaves seem to work only fresh, not when dried and should be frozen for extended storage. Quite a few leaves (50 or so) are required for a trip.

CALIFORNIA POPPY

This versatile plant is grown as an annual in cold areas and as a perennial in warmer climates. It is an herb which attains heights in the two foot region, favors sun and rocky soils, and should be started where it is going to grow as it does not transplant too well.

The leaves, flowers, and seed pods are all good.

These are the most common do-it-yourself highs, but almost any organic plant, including kava kava, yage, etc. could be grown. Some of the books listed in the further reading list get into this sort of thing on a more extensive level.

SUPPLIERS

The following companies carry some seeds, cuttings, plants, or supplies of interest to the person experimenting with organic psychotropic drugs. However, they are, almost without exception, straight companies doing business with the general public, so don't ask a lot of funny questions. . .

If you are going to order a catalog be sure to include at least 25 cents for postage and handling (unless otherwise indicated.)

Electric Earth Herbs — Box 261, Sonora, California 95370. Stocks San Pedro Cactus, hip oriented, they know why you want it. . .

R.C. Seed Company — Box 361, Redwood City, California 94061. Seeds.

George Park Seed Company — Greenwood, South Carolina 29646. Seeds.

Burpee Seed Company — 6450 Rutland, Riverside, California 92502.

New Mexico Cactus Research Company — Box 787, Belen, New Mexico. Cacti offspring.

Wine and the People — 1140 University Avenue, Berkeley, California. Hops and hop supplies.

Magic Garden Herb Company — Box 332, Fairfax, California. Various herbs, including Yohimbe, Broom, Kava Kava.

Stackhouse — Box 1262, Southgate, Michigan 48195. Lactose and pure lab chemicals.

Columbia Organic Chemicals — 912 Drake Street, Columbia, South Carolina. Yohimbe, etc.

Karma Kem Ko — Box 235, Yatesboro, Pennsylvania 16263. Name should be fairly self-explanatory. . .

Mathesid-Coleman-Bell — Box 1622, Milwaukee, Wisconsin.

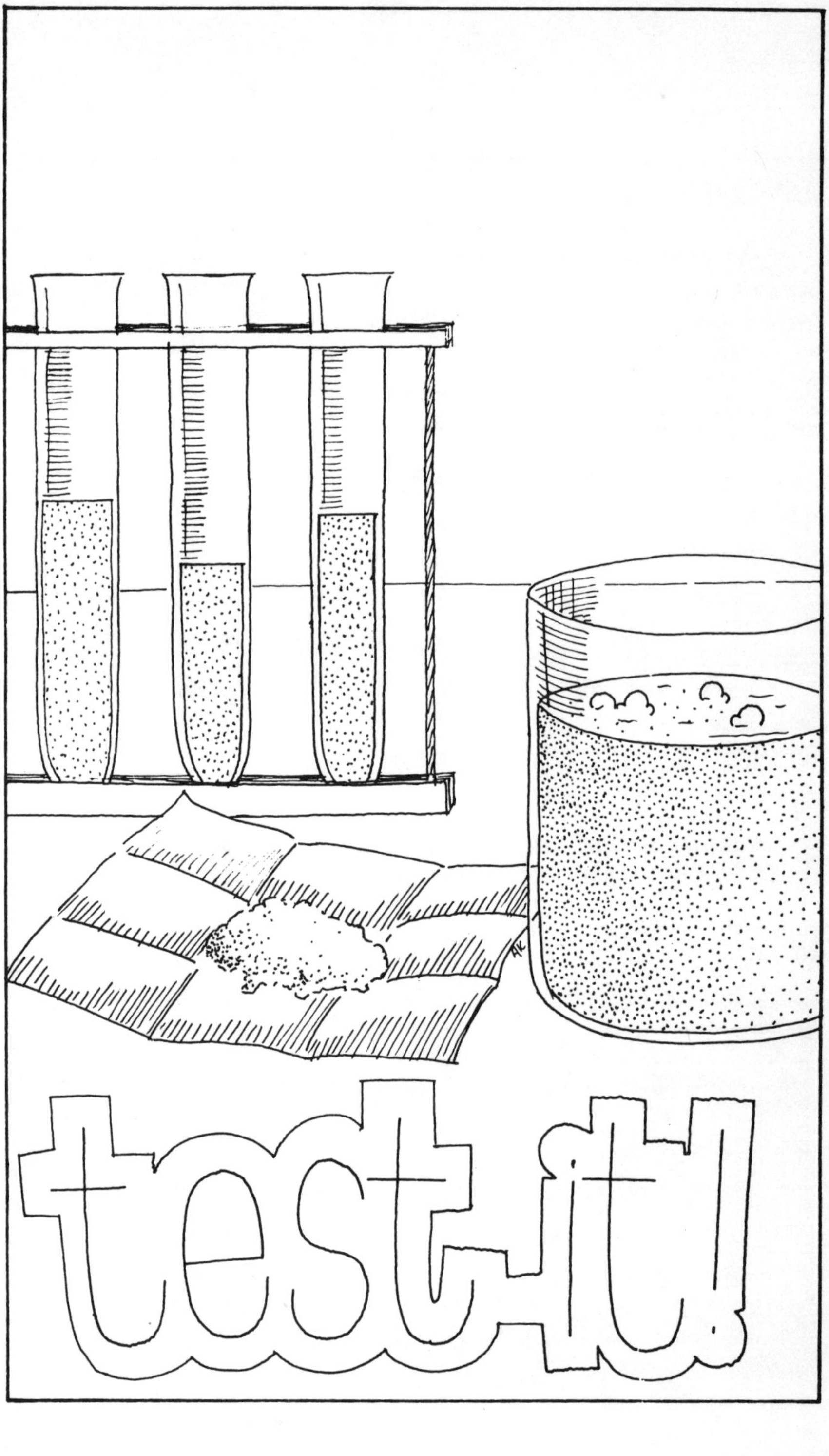
test it!

TEST IT!

There are a number of simple chemical tests that can be run on any drug or suspected drug sample. In each case, the chemicals may be purchased relatively inexpensively and without prescription, special license, or trouble.

Unless otherwise stated, a small bit of the suspect material will suffice, usually about the size of a match head. In tests where more than one chemical is required one should be sure all chemicals are used in equal amounts.

The chemicals are dangerous if mishandled. Don't attempt to conduct the test while stoned, don't allow the chemicals around anyone who is likely to be irresponsible with them. If any of the acids are spilled on skin or clothing, you should wash the affected area in cold water and then baking soda. If formaldehyde, methyl or ethyl alcohol, chloroform are swallowed, try to induce vomiting and call a physician. If the acids are swallowed, DO NOT induce vomiting, but call a physician and the victim should be given milk or milk of magnesia.

After each test, the test tube, plate, or whatever must be flushed clean with baking soda and water and running water to prevent any contamination in the next test.

If a suspect gives a positive reaction, you can be reasonably assured it is what it is purported to be. However, this does NOT indicate it is not adulterated with something else, just that it is present. If you have a confirming result, you can retest (another sample) with the other tests to discover any adulterants.

A quick result coupled with a deep or dark positive color may indicate a relatively potent concentration of the test material, BUT this is not foolproof, due to variables in conditions, reactions, and adulterants.

Keep all chemicals tightly closed. A series of tests in already bottled form, for some of the following tests may be purchased through Western Scientific Products, 5424 Vineland Avenue, North Hollywood, California 91601.

BARBITURATES

Testing:

Two reagents should be employed here: first isoproylamine and then cobalt acetate dissolved in methyl alcohol.

Secobarbital will turn this mixture a reddish purple. Normal tranquilizers and pain-killers will be unaffected by this test.

COCAINE

Testing:

Coke is normally tested by adding about four drops of cobalt thiocyanate. If positive, a dark blue, flaky precipitate will form. If the entire material turns blue right away, it is relatively potent. If dark blue flecks appear right after adding the chemical and then the whole material turns blue, it is probably adulterated, with the primary dark spots being the coke.

Unfortunately procaine, which will not get you high, also tests out blue with this test.

Once you ascertain that the substance is coke, some value judgment can be passed by physical examination, taste, and the burning test.

Flake coke (the form pharmaceuticals come in) is the hardest to adulterate, as the common adulterants are in powder or crystal form. Rock is semisafe, BUT the rocks can be dissolved and reformed with little hassle to give the appearance of purity.

Coke is often cut with local anesthetics such as procaine, benzocaine, etc., as well as with lactose, speed, and epsom salts.

Lactose leaves a sweetish taste if eaten, salt is dull and usually has the characteristic salt taste. Epsom salts are grainy and quite sour in taste. The local anesthetics such as procaine numb the face sooner after ingestion and feel much like what is experienced in a dentist's chair. Local anesthetics give no high, so if the numbing is quite pronounced, and the high is minimal, you are using more anesthetic than anything else.

A small sample can be put in a spoon and heated over an alcohol burner or even a match. Pure coke burns clear and leaves no residue. Refined coke burns just a trifle brownish and leaves a small bit of ash. Anything else mixed in with the coke will leave behind some telltale sign in direct proportion to its strength: sugar leaves a black carbon ash; salts will not burn and remain behind; speed pops with a crackling sound; local anesthetics cause the mixture to bubble in burning.

If you feel speed has been used as a cut, test with the amphetamine test (which will not be affected by coke).

CODEINE

Codeine is a fairly cheap, somewhat stony drug that is used to cut coke, smack, and even speed.

Four drops of concentrated sulfuric acid will turn codeine blue-green.

Or:

Mix the suspect with four drops of formalin, a 30 per cent formaldehyde solution, should give a purple flash and then go colorless.

Or:

Mix .05 gram of suspect with 2 cc of concentrated nitric acid. If a yellow appears and remains, it is codeine.

HASH

Same test procedures as marijuana. Hash is rarely cut with anything, but may vary in strength according to the grades, countries, crop, etc. (see hash section). A more likely ploy for a hash rip-off is to use part of a real brick (or ball, etc.) of high grade hash and fill the center with cork, and other inert materials.

HEROIN

All street heroin is cut. The major problem in heroin is not receiving a cut dose (of say 1-6 per cent), but in getting a potent dose by mistake and overdosing on a normal hit.

Smack used to be cut primarily with quinine, which gave it a bitter taste that many users think indicates the presence of heroin. In actuality, heroin is almost tasteless.

Today, most smack is cut with lactose, so the bitter-taste-test does not apply.

Heroin will turn a yellow which gradually changes to a green-blue when added to a few drops of concentrated nitric acid.

Or:

Four drops of concentrated sulfuric acid will turn heroin green.

LSD

Testing:

Combine a small sample of suspect material with four drops of di-methyl-benzaldehyde and add concentrated hydrochloric acid drop by drop. DO NOT USE MORE THAN FIVE DROPS. If acid is present, the material will turn lavender.

If PCP is present in the acid, it will give a yellow reaction, BUT this is not positive as other substances may also cause it to react in this manner.

LSD is made and then tasted. Someone eats a bit to see what the reaction is. If the acid is nice and the trip is fairly mellow, it will be packaged as acid and sold as such.

If the high is strange, that is, weird side effects, it will probably be mixed with PCP and sold as some exotic drug (mesc., psilocybin, MDA, etc., etc.,).

Another test is called the chloroform extraction test: take about four drops of acetaldehyde, vanillin, and ethyl and methyl alcohol (all one mixture) and mix with the sample. Shake for about fifteen seconds and add a similar amount of concentrated hydrochloric acid. If a purple color forms, you then add half an inch of chloroform to the test vial, cap it, and shake again for fifteen seconds. If the purple color refuses to leave the top layer and mix with the chloroform, it is positively LSD.

MARIJUANA

Many people assume that their grass had been adulterated with some weird thing because of all the PCP floating around. In actuality very little marijuana is ever treated with PCP (although parsley, oregano, mint, etc., is and sold as grass or "superweed," etc.). Accidently, a number of other weeds may have been cut with your grass and may cause an unusual reddening of the eyes or stinging sensation. If you have been drinking alcohol, expect the classic "spinning" sensation, which can also indicate adulteration.

If your grass has been treated, you should notice a strong chemical smell in the first hit or two.

Recognizing Weeds:

When a social user of grass is exposed to dynamite shit, he may experience an intense reaction, which can lead to paranoia and the fear that he has just used smacked, opiated or DMTed grass. Usually this fear is groundless, but heightened by severe stone and the paranoia, it becomes quite real. About 60 per cent (or more) of the weed sold in the U.S. is of the homegrown variety and is usually weaker in strength than the imported types.

American weed is usually a more greenish color than Mexican which is gold or brown. Panama comes in the familiar "red" tint, while African or Far Eastern may be almost black.

Often a Mexican connection will put coca cola over grass which doesn't have enough surface resin to effective stick in a brick shape. Run your finger (wet) over the brick and taste it to see if it has the sugary sweet taste which coke (not the real thing, in this case) imparts to grass. Too much coke or sugar water makes the grass very harsh to smoke, throws in all sorts of strange chemicals, increases the weight of the kilo without adding more weed, and can very likely indicate poor quality grass.

Of course, the best way to test the quality is to smoke a joint which YOU take from the brick. If the brick is packaged and one end is torn open, get your sample from the opposite end.

Testing:

The government uses a test known as the Duquesnois test to indicate the presence of THC (hence grass and hash). This test will also react positively to the sterile hemp seed in canary feed, but the government uses it anyway.

Mix a small amount with acetaldehyde, vanillin (can be dissolved in alcohol), wait about fifteen seconds and add an equal amount of concentrated hydrochloric acid. If THC is present, a blue to blue-violet will appear.

If the above result is positive, you can add about ½ inch of chloroform to the vial, cap it, and shake. Let settle. If the blue color is taken out and goes into the chloroform layer, it is positive. This test will work on ashes or vegetable matter.

For Adulterants: Lower quality grass is sometimes adulterated with other chemicals to improve its market value. Any of the various tests in this chapter will work with marijuana to show you if this holds true for your sample.

A wide band adulterant test is to take the grass and vigorously scrub it in a small dish of water. The THC will not go into solution, but many chemicals will (especially those which have been dusted on).

To your wash water add a few drops of ferric chloride. If a red color appears, you can be fairly sure that the grass has been treated with a no-no.

If the red color is present, heat the test tube over a light heat. If the red disappears, it probably was not an opiate, and you should start with another sample and test for other possibilities.

Take another tube full of wash water and add a few drops of lead acetate in alcohol. If opium is present, a white precipitate will appear and remain. If a few drops of nitric acid are added, this white will disappear.

Low grade opium and wasted morphine (a by-product of smack manufacture) are often used to adulterate grass, but occasionally, PCP, barbiturates and even speed will appear.

Very seldom will you find DMT, heroin, etc. used as their market value exceeds that of the grass being treated.

A less specific test for THC is to add a bit of suspect to 5 per cent KOH in ethanol. A red color is positive.

PCP

PCP will turn the combination of dimethylaminobenzaldehyde and HCL used in the LSD test to a yellow. However, there may possibly be other substances that will also produce this yellow reaction.

PSILOCYBIN

Always consult a good mushroom book before attempting to use any of the psilocybin family! Real psilocybin mushrooms are bitter tasting and require more than one mushroom to get you off (unlike the LSD-spiked common mushrooms sold as Psilocybin).

Testing:

A true psilocybin mushroom will bruise to a blue or bluish tint. (This will not work on dried mushrooms). A more positive ID can be obtained by using methaminophenol sulphate, which can be purchased under the trade name Pictol from photo supply houses.

Take a small quantity of Pictol and add it to about 20 times its own weight in distilled water. Right then apply the solution to the suspected mushroom (on the stem) and wait. Within a half hour, a deep purple color should appear on the treated portion of the fungi, if it is indeed psilocybin.

Synthetic psilocybin is available as a powder or liquid and has be been found in both caps and in tablets. Average does is 20 – 60 milligrams, but may run many times that.

About one in every 1,000 – 2,000 samples of suspected psilocybin is the real thing on the street.

COMMERCIAL ANALYSIS

PharmChem: 1848 Bay Road, Palo Alto, California 94303 will analyze any sample drug mailed in for a fee of $10 and will give results by phone (415) 322-9941 three days after the sample is received. One can preserve one's identity if one so wishes by giving any five-digit number to the sample and giving only this number when one calls.

They would like to know what you think the sample is, where you got it, and what the street price is/was.

D.C. Free Clinic: 1556 Wisconsin Avenue, Washington, D.C., 965-5976. Free drug analyzing with the number bit so no name comes into play.

130. LSD	LSD	blue tablet, 1/16" diam. x 1/32"
131. LSD	LSD	brown double-dome tablet, 1/4" diam. x 5/32"
132. LSD	LSD	light purple tablet, 1/4" diam. x 1/8"
133. LSD	LSD	orange tablet, broken
134. LSD	LSD	dark brown gelatin square, 3/32" x 3/32"
135. LSD	LSD	blue tablet, 1/16" diam. x 1/32"
136. LSD	LSD	blue-violet tablet, 3/16" diam. x 3/32"
137. LSD	LSD	orange spot on white blotter paper with red & blue design
138. LSD	LSD	blue-green spot on white blotter paper with red & blue design
139. LSD	LSD	amber gelatin square, 3/32" x 3/32", "Clearlight"
140. LSD	no drug detected	white blotter paper
141. LSD	no drug detected	blue spot on white blotter paper, "150ug"
142. Marijuana	marijuana	green-brown plant material & seeds
143. Marijuana	marijuana	green plant material, "Maui"
144. Marijuana	marijuana	green plant material & seeds
145. Marijuana	marijuana	green-brown plant material & seeds
146. Marijuana	marijuana	green-brown plant material
147. Marijuana	marijuana	green-brown plant material
148. Marijuana	marijuana	green plant material
149. Marijuana	marijuana	green plant material & seeds
150. Marijuana	marijuana	green-brown plant material & seeds
151. Marijuana	marijuana	green plant material
152. Marijuana	marijuana	green plant material & seeds
153. Marijuana	marijuana	green plant material & seeds, "Michoachan"
154. Marijuana	marijuana	green plant material & seeds
155. Marijuana	marijuana	green plant material
156. Marijuana	no drug detected	green plant material & stems
157. Mescaline	mescaline + other alkaloids of Lophophora williamsii	brown powder in pink papsule
158. Mescaline	LSD	white powder
159. Mescaline	LSD	light brown powder in clear capsule, 23/32" x 1/4"
160. Mescaline	LSD + iso-LSD	yellow tablet, 3/32" diam. x 1/16"
161. Mescaline	LSD	white powder in clear capsule, 3/4" x 1/4"
162. Mescaline	LSD	white powder in clear capsule
163. Mescaline	LSD	brown tablet, 1/4" diam. x 1/16"
164. Mescaline	LSD + PCP	red-brown tablet, 1/4" diam. x 1/8"
165. Mescaline	PCP	white powder in clear capsule, 13/16" x 9/32"
166. Mescaline	methamphetamine	white powder
167. Mescaline	no drug detected	white powder
168. Methamphetamine	caffeine	cross-scored white tablet, 1/4" diam. x 1/16"
169. Methamphetamine	ephedrine + caffeine	scored white tablet, 1/4" diam. x 3/32"
170. Methaqualone	ephedrine + phenobarbital + theophylline	scored white tablet, 7/16" diam. x 5/32"
171. Methaqualone	promethazine	white powder in blue & turquoise capsule
172. Opium	opium + morphine + codeine	dark brown brittle solid
173. Opium	no drug detected	black brittle solid
174. Opium	no drug detected	black amorphous solid
175. Opium	no drug detected	black brittle solid
176. PCP	PCP + mint leaves	green plant material
177. Psilocybin	LSD	light brown tablet, 1/4" diam. x 1/8"
178. Psilocybin	LSD	brown mushroom slices
179. Psilocybin	LSD	brown mushroom pieces
180. Psilocybin	LSD	dried mushroom pieces
181. Psilocybin	LSD	brown mushroom pieces
182. Psilocybin	LSD	dried brown mushroom piece
183. Psilocybin	mescaline + other alkaloids of Lophophora williamsii	dried brown plant material
184. Secobarbital	phenobarbital	clear liquid
185. THC	PCP	"salt & pepper" powder
186. THC	PCP	off-white powder, "TIC"
187. ?	phenylpropanolamine + chlorpheniramine + methapyriline	scored turquoise tablet, 13/32" x 5/32"
188. ?	imipramine	white powder in pink capsule, 9/16" x 3/16"
189. ?	amobarbital + secobarbital	white powder
190. ?	imipramine	orange-coated tablet, 7/32" diam. x 1/8"
191. ?	strychnine	white powder
192. ?	marijuana	olive-drab plant material & seeds
193. ?	heroin	grey-brown powder in clear capsule, 15/16" x 5/16'
194. ?	1-[1-(2-thiophenyl)cyclohexyl] piperidine	white powder
195. ?	propoxyphene	white granular powder

A partial look at one month's analysis results from PharmChem Labs. Notice the similarity of alleged content versus actual content in both PharmChem's findings and our own. . .

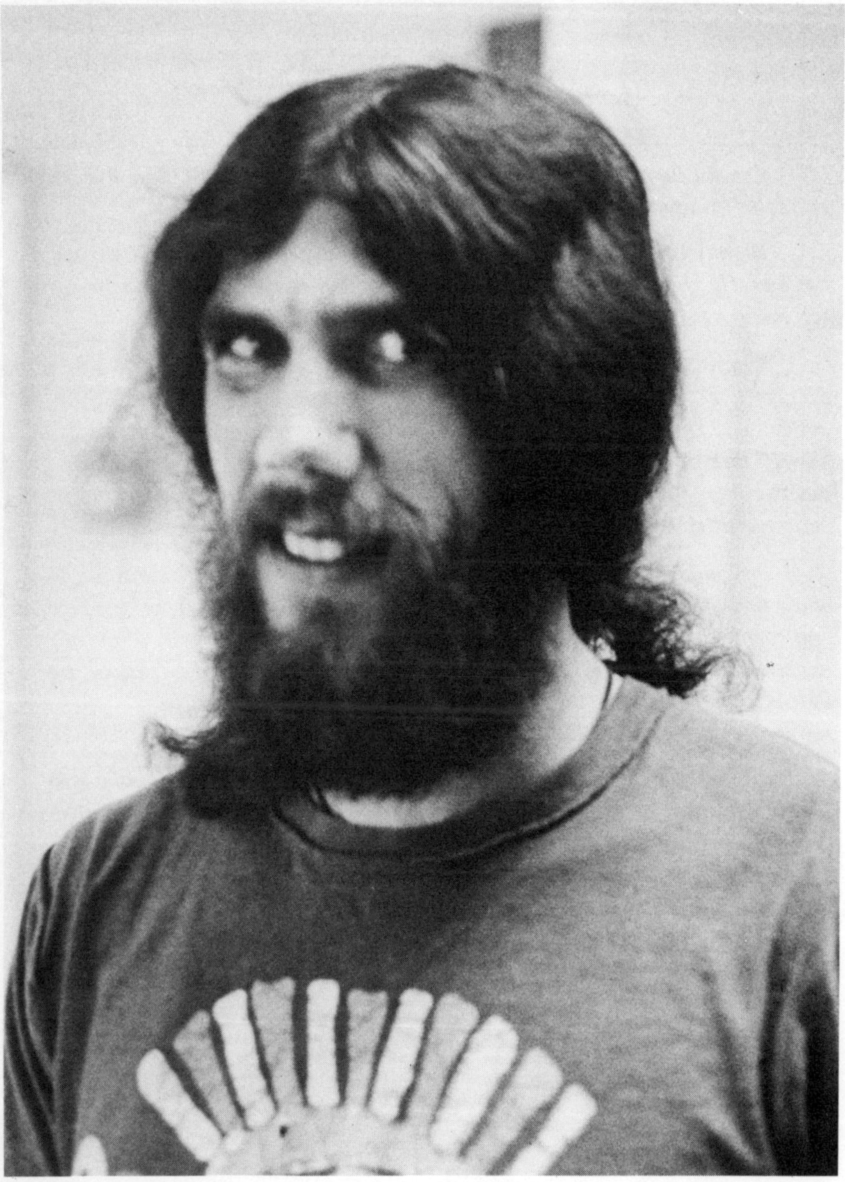

Bruce Ratcliffe, Ph.D., driving force behind one of the largest and best organized drug analzying laboratories in the U.S., PharmChem Laboratories in Palo Alto, California.

PharmChem Labs in Palo Alto, California is one of the oldest and best equipped anonymous drug testing laboratories in the country.

Organized over two years ago as a non-profit entity, PharmChem also has a profit oriented sister company which analyzes such things as urine samples for traces of drugs.

PharmChem employs four people and performs about thirty-five tests in an average week. Each drug that is submitted to PharmChem (from the Bay Area and all over the country) undergoes a sophisticated testing program consisting of 10 - 15 tests to determine exactly what and what quantity. The results are given out to callers (as described herein) as well as being published in a weekly publication entitled the Friday Drug News.

Periodically, the administration will "crack down" on labs and refuse to allow them to issue quantitative reports, on the thought that neferious pushers and chemists are using the labs for reports on their own products (PharmChem experienced such a crackdown soon after the formation of the D.E.A.), but as this is being written, they are allowed to issue both, qualitative and quantitative, reports and will do so for $5.00 and $10.00 respectively.

PharmChem has analyzed samples of just about everything under the proverbial sun from oregano to household cleanser, and reported such diverse drugs as Scopalamine (from Arizona) and even a tablet of Ibogaine (this one all the way from Paris.)

The following is a chart showing the results of 14 months (72-72) of street drug identification. The samples were taken from all sectors of the U.S.

Alleged Content	Real Content							
	MES	LSD	Lsd/Pcp	PCP	THC	AMP	Other	Number
Mesc	13	198	34				23	268
LSD		403	11				48	462
Psil	1	87	18	6			4	119
Amp		3				166	36	205
THC			4	79			19	102
STP		16	5			23 (STP)	4	48
TOTALS	14	707	72	85	0	189	134	1204

Others: Samples of opiates tested usually were opiates, although of lower quality and cut. Several were only codeine, a couple were saccharin, and two samples of "opium" were black incense.

Grass was usually grass, occasionally treated. Hash was hash 19 times out of 20, but the percentage of THC varied greatly.

DRUG ANALYSIS SAMPLE

Alleged Content	Real Content	Description	Filler (if any)
Mescaline	LSD	brown powder	sugar/lactose/ chocolate
Mescaline	LSD/PCP	brown speckled tab	stearic acid
Mescaline	Mescaline	white powder	?
LSD	LSD	orange tab	sugar
LSD	LSD/PCP	green tab	stearic acid
Psilocybin	LSD	brown powder cap	yeast
Psilocybin	LSD/PCP	pink powder	?
MDA	MDA	white powder	sugar
Cocaine	Cocaine	white powder	procaine
THC	PCP	white tab	sugar
Peyote root	couldn't identify	brown root pieces	?
Speed w/mescaline	LSD	brown powder	?
Chocolate mescaline	LSD	brown powder	chocolate
Syn mescaline	LSD	lrg white cap	flour

BUMMERS AND WIPEOUT

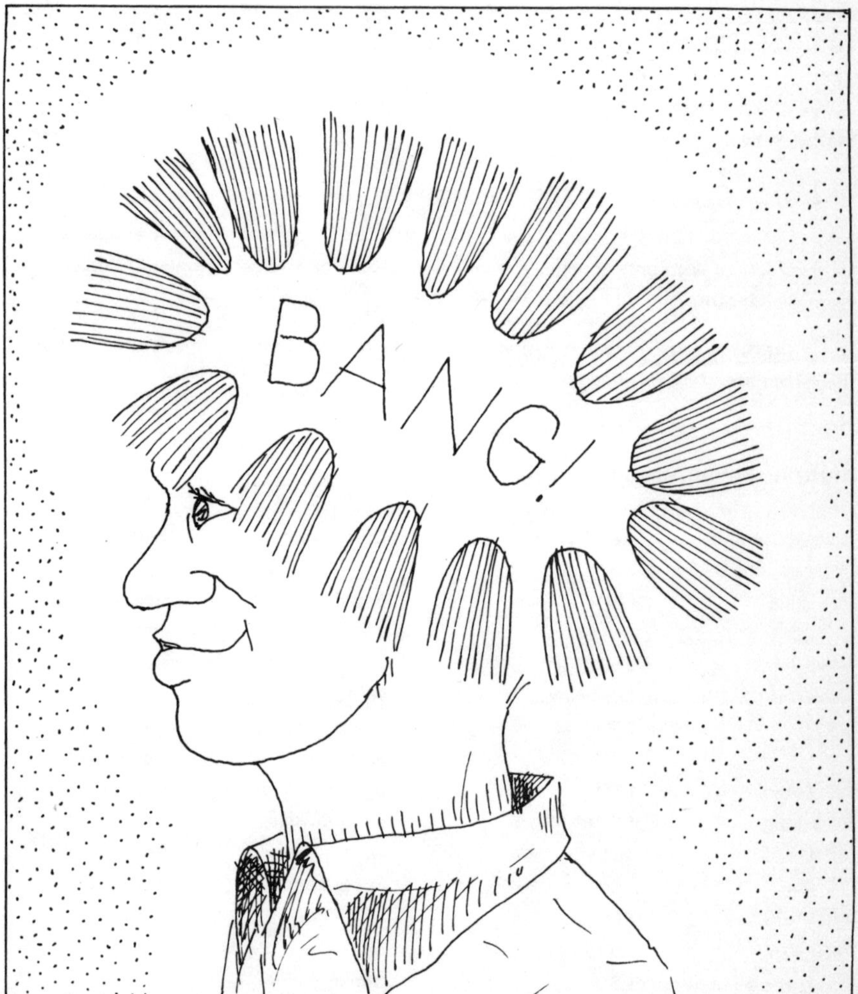

BUMMERS AND WIPEOUT

LSD

Bummers: An acid trip seems to be either spectacular or bad. There is little middle ground. A good trip usually makes the user feel like he is secure, on top of the world, as well as tuned in to his surroundings and to other people to an extraordinary degree.

On the other hand, a bummer can set off a spiraling reaction of bad thoughts and uncontrollable emotions in the user. Horrible thoughts and experiences may build up one on the other. This can be triggered by an outside experience or by the user's own thoughts as well as by the quality of the drug.

Some batches of a certain drug seem high quality, pure, and about the right dosage. This drug may have very few to no bad trips, while other batches may be very lacking in quality control, or mixed with some other drug to amplify their effects and may cause consistent bad times. Besides the drug itself, three things are generally thought to have an appreciable effect on the contents of the trip:

1. A good "set." This translates as a pleasant frame of mind, free of fear or heavy side trips about personal things.

2. Environment. This should be steady and relaxed, hopefully the type of surroundings the user can identify with. Excess people, confusing sounds, and extraneous noise, can lead to problems.

3. A guide. Especially when dealing with novices, a good trip guide can be invaluable.

The fear of being busted is a major cause of bad trips. LSD can amplify emotions to an unreal degree that seems perfectly normal in the user. Persons who are called upon to level a bummer must be aware of this fact. This is especially true if anyone in authority is present, i.e., doctors, police, parents, ministers, etc. The person tending the tripper must make a decision whether to cope alone or call in someone of authority.

If it is a medical emergency of any kind, downer overdose and bodily symptoms, a doctor must be called. To not do so means you are killing someone — always.

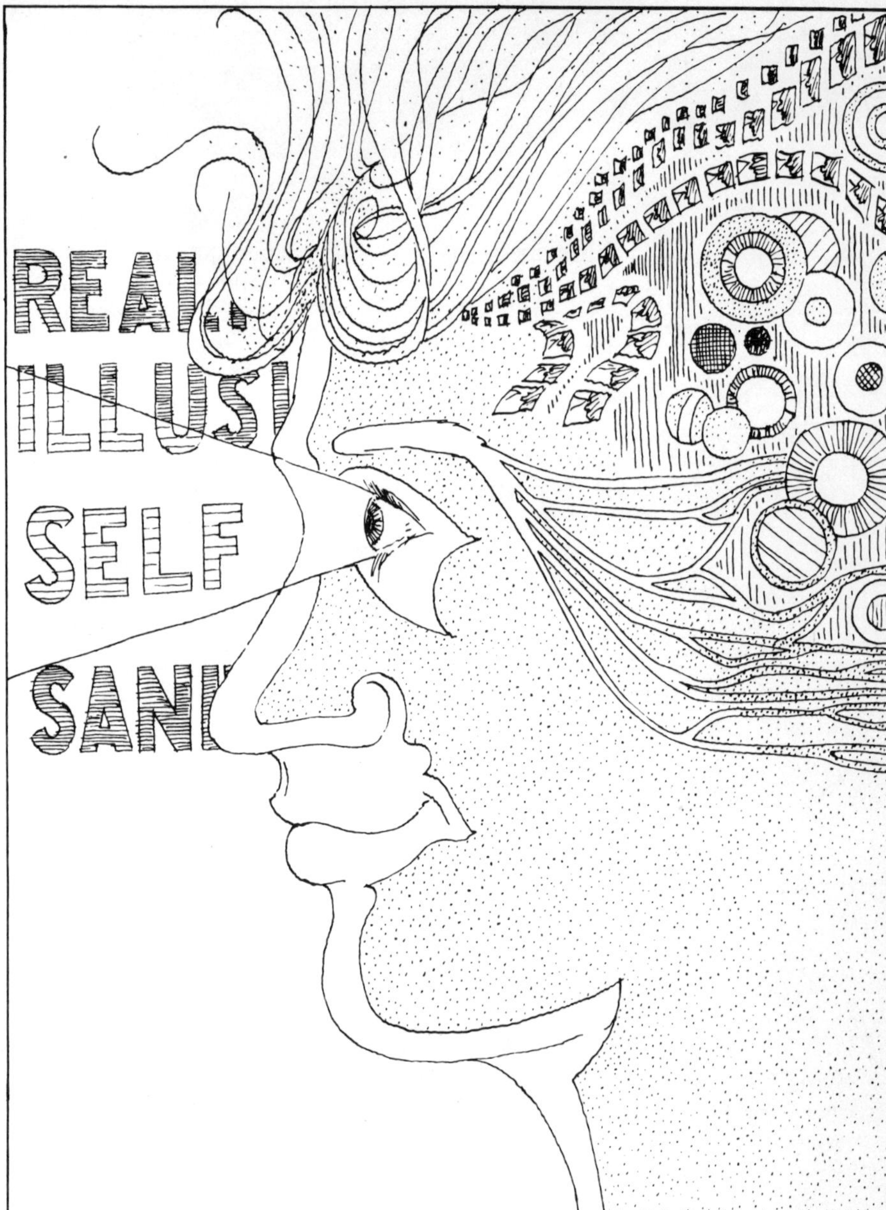
REAL
ILLUS
SELF
SAN

However, in a psychedelic bummer, a person in a uniform can often heighten the user's paranoia to an unconquerable degree. Also, you must realize there are many unsympathetic people who do not have the training to deal with this situation including many doctors.

If you have done drugs you can probably get a better picture of the person's state than a straight helper. Occasionally going to a hospital for help means he is strait-jacketed and left to suffer or shot up with thorazine and sent to the mental ward.

Mental wards and jails are not the best places to find yourself in when freaking out.

If a person in authority is called it is often best to have him work through a third party, usually someone the user knows and trusts.

TREATING THE FREAK OUT

Physiological treatment: Normal LSD is treated by administering thorazine. However, this is not recommended for home use—thorazine tends to produce a bad reaction when mixed with PCP and a percentage of the acid on the streets does have some PCP mixed in.

There is also the possibility of thorazine reacting badly with plain LSD. All in all, it is not an amateur treatment. Niacin (vitamin B_3) helps bring the user down and smooths out the rest of the trip somewhat.

Psychological treatment: With psychotropic drugs and unlike most other drugs, the psychological treatment is usually the most important and effective treatment.

A bad trip often begins with the user exhibiting signs of fear or nervousness. Do not underestimate this signal, but remain calm and suggest everything will mellow out soon and he should try to ride it out. Always tell him you'll be there to help if anything gets bad. NEVER ATTEMPT TO GO INTO EXTENSIVE QUESTIONING ABOUT THE BAD REACTIONS! It is not a good thing to say such things as, "Gee, that sounds like that bad acid all those people freaked out on."

Do not attempt to control the person, rather take your clues from him and guide him. A complete trust factor is very necessary to help him at all.

It may be helpful to ask the person concrete (who are you, where are we) kinds of questions about himself and his activities that DO NOT have anything to do with the bad trip. This is expecially helpful whenever the user gets the paranoia that the trip will never end, or he has done permanent damage to himself and will not recover.

He may scream or wish to go to a better place (whether physically or mentally) where he can better control his anxieties. This is especially true if he is around a group of people and feels humiliated about losing control. This is a common reaction which must be nullified by the guide.

It is sometimes a good idea to move the person to a quiet place where he is not apt to feel self-conscious and can relax to some degree.

It may be helpful to touch the person, IF HE WANTS IT, as it may establish a personal warmth. Humor can help if the user feels he is laughing WITH you and not the object of the humor.

If the person gets very heavily into a paranoia thing, you must remember he is in a state of very increased awareness and probably has some very real things to be paranoid about.

Don't tell him his fears are foolish, try to understand his situation and help him out of it. If the tripper makes it obvious that his problems are strictly internal, the best approach is just to establish warmth and security by assuring him that you'll stay and help him out and that he is going to be all right. However, his fears will probably last throughout the entire trip and may remain valid for some time afterwards.

Remember, reestablish concrete things (I'm Bill and you're Bob, and I'm going to stay with you, and everything will be okay). Repeat this over and over. If any tactic seems to be working – stay with it. If he doesn't react, switch to something else. If the tripper becomes totally incoherent or very violent and appears to be capable of damaging himself or others – get him to an emergency ward.

It is nice to keep an emergency list of crisis centers and hospitals that are known to be cool – a hospital does not have to report trippers, although some will. You are in no trouble, you don't know how he got the drug, etc., you're just trying to help him.

WIPEOUT

Drug wipeout is a real, physiological condition, evolving from overuse of drugs within a specific period or even from a single, severe, and probably bad trip. It is a feeling most chronic users have probably experienced, or are experiencing and is characterized by the vague, uneasy feeling, wanting to do things, but not being able to "get it together," occasional flashback of some sort or another, loss of memory and the "blahs" — a physical blah feeling sometimes felt in the inner neck and back of the head region.

Wipeout can cause a distinct problem in correlating the thought patterns with the physical action of speech. A user may be able to think fine, but when he tries to communicate, there is no coordination between the mind and speech organs. This leads to frustration and fear that some permanent damage has been done.

Often the wipeout case becomes schizo-upset and irritated by little things that would normally not bother him. He may be very frightened inside. This condition has led to a number of suicides, including one good friend of the author's.

There is a positive, reliable treatment for the drug wipeout which seems to work in over 90 per cent of the cases tried. It is known as megavitamin therapy, and consists of the victim taking large amounts of vitamin C and Niacin (B_3).

About 2,000 mg. of the drugs are taken orally every day. This is best accomplished at mealtimes and can be spread out over the day.

The user may experience a heat flash reaction about a half hour after ingesting the Niacin. This is a natural bodily reaction to the drug and is not harmful. It will pass shortly.

Within two weeks all symptoms of the drug wipeout should have disappeared and the user should be back to "normal." This treatment is being used successfully in treating clinical schizophrenics also.

DOWNERS – ODs

ODs are probably the most dangerous type of drug-related emergency. They are also the worst to treat or make decisions about treating. This is especially true on strong downers where you can expect the person to nod out a bit.

REMEMBER — depressants make a person superrelaxed, but, he should still be able to be aroused. If not, he's in trouble.

ODs happen because the bloodstream becomes overloaded with a drug (or drugs) and the bodily organs can no longer cope with the high concentration. Some drugs, like phenobarbital, can take over an hour to come on, so the user will redrop before he is off, and the next batch won't catch up for a while.

A person suffering from downer overdose will lapse into unconsciousness, draw shallow breaths and generally have trouble breathing, and may die if he doesn't get help.

Try and get the person moving, walk him around the room, supporting him if necessary. Slap his face repeatedly. If his breathing stops at any point, immediately give artificial respiration, and GET HIM TO A HOSPITAL. Death can occur in minutes.

Shooting a person full of salt, uppers, etc., mainly wastes time and does not increase his survival chances.

Do not induce vomiting unless the person is QUITE alert. In most cases, vomiting is only effective for about fifteen minutes after the person takes the pills. If he has shot up anything, vomiting doesn't help at all. If the person is lapsing into unconsciousness and you induce vomiting, it may clog his windpipe and choke him to death.

If a person is dying, you must take the responsibility and ACT. Being high yourself and debating the "we'll-have-to-face-the-doctors-and-all-those-bright-lights" trip may kill your friend. GET HIM TO A HOSPITAL.

Another interesting point is guilt reaction. You should never have to feel guilty about taking anyone for treatment. After the person recovers, he may feel very bad about his role and go into the "I would have been all right if you'd just left me along" thing. BULLSHIT! You probably saved the idiot's life. You don't have to apologize for it!

UPPER OD

While there are clinical overdose potentials with uppers, they are usually not so easily reached as with downers. The person who ODs on speed or coke will feel very paranoid and, needless to say, rushed.

He may be so wired, he grits his teeth and cannot move, with his heart beating so fast he thinks he is going to die. The psychological treatment is much like with psychotropic drugs — convince him it will pass and that you'll help him through the bad periods.

Giving tranquilizers is not recommended. The feeling will pass anywhere from fifteen minutes to two hours from the initial paranoia.

Physiological: Niacin (B_3) seems to help bring down the

user somewhat, and milk helps to even it out.

The megavitamin treatment is useful for the speed user-abuser, also, as the niacin tends to purge the bloodstream of impurities, and the vitamin C helps put a little joy back into your step. Of course, this should be used with a balanced diet and other vitamin supplements to avoid overbalancing the body any worse than it already is.

COCAINE OVERDOSE

This is all but impossible (well, nothing is impossible for the really determined, but it is hard), unless the drug is injected.

Should this occur, follow the rules for any overdose which produces passing out and stoppage of breathing, including artificial respiration and heart massage.

For partial ODs (by snorting or eating), wash the stomach out with sodium bicarbonate and warm water. If faint, inhale ammonia.

BELLADONNA OVERDOSE

This is a rare and hard to diagnose condition. Belladonna has the nasty habit of causing the user to see very real-appearing snakes, bugs, germs, and spiders along with a generally rotten trip, so it is hard to tell an overdose.

However, if the patient becomes violent or catatonic or lapses into unconsciousness, he should be taken to a physician and treated with atropine which counteracts the condition.

WITHDRAWAL

Withdrawal is a bodily reaction (or set of reactions) signaling the body's need for more depressants. It can occur with any number of downers from heroin to Quaalude. The symptoms include:

yawning
running nose
muscle twitching
chills
anziety
dizziness
diarrhea
stomach pain, etc.

Heroin withdrawal is a bitch, but barbiturate and Quaalude withdrawal can easily KILL you. Go to a hospital.

HEPATITIS

There are two types of hepatitis: infectious and serum.

Infectious is thought to be contracted from fecal contamination, contact, contaminated water supplies, and sometimes from shellfish raised in contaminated waters.

Serum hepatitis is most easily transmitted through blood or blood product transfusions, contaminated needles and syringes.

Hepatitis shows up in symptoms much like the flu: weakness, fatigue, sweatiness, depression, possibly loss of appetite, and stomach disorder.

The liver is tender and may enlarge, the patient becomes crabby and may develop acnelike rashes.

When jaundice is present (the yellow skin/eyes and urine), the disease is most easily found. Jaundice usually peaks about two weeks into the disease and then recedes over the next two - six weeks, but about 15 - 20 per cent will suffer a relapse.

The treatment of hepatitis is lots of rest and a high protein diet. The patient may develop weird appetites and should be encouraged to eat whatever and whenever he desires. High calorie foods are also good. At no time can the patient have alcohol or unprescribed drugs of any kind as the liver is already overworked to the breaking point.

Go to a physician. Other members of the household can get preventive gamma globulin shots and should avoid ANY contact with the patient's dishes, glasses, needles, or personal items.

Hep can stay in the blood for several YEARS after the symptoms, possibly even for a lifetime. For this reason, you should NEVER allow another human to come in contact with needles you have used after contacting hep.

IMBIBING

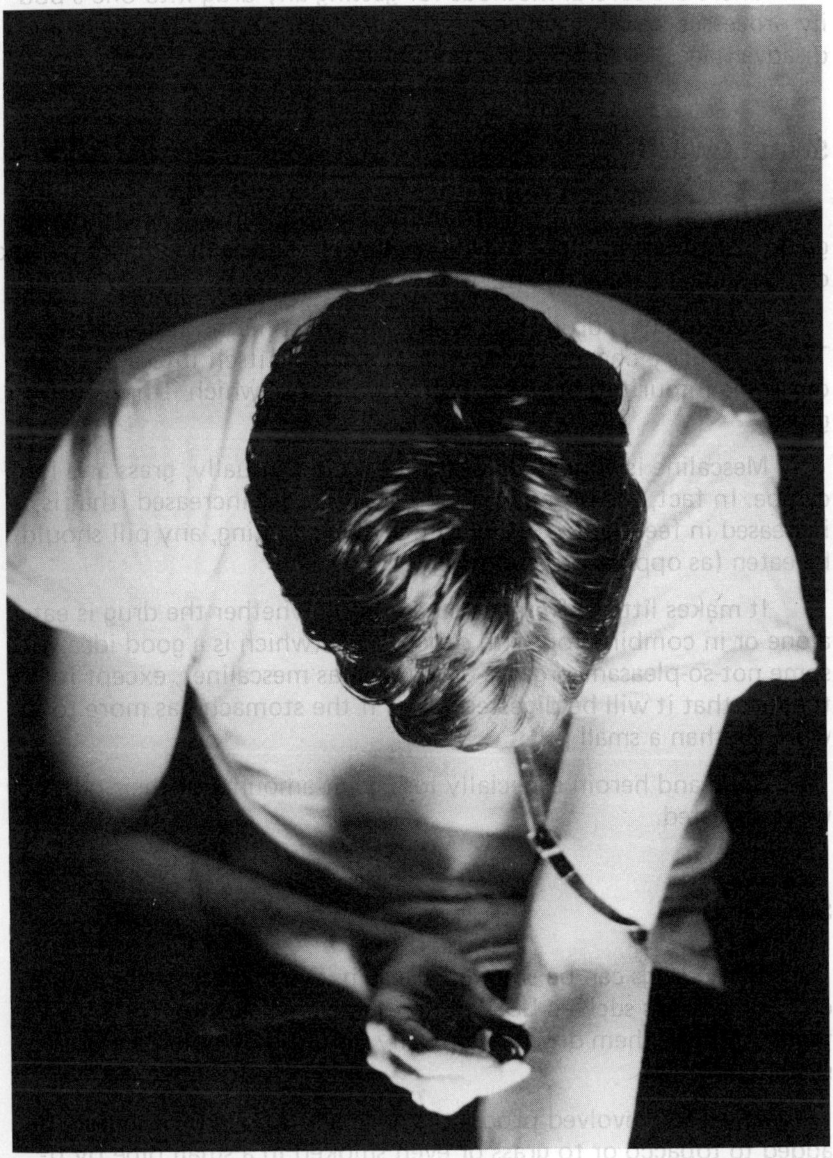

IMBIBING

There are several methods for getting any drug into one's bodily processes, each of which has its particular set of advantages and disadvantages.

SWALLOWING

This is the common method for any pill, capsule, and most organic plant matter. Most LSD is swallowed, although almost any acid can be shot if care is taken.

Swallowing a drug is generally the safest method of ingestion. The body has a chance to see what it's getting itself into and filter out some impurities or reject (vomit up) those which it finds too gross.

Mescaline is almost always eaten, acid is usually, grass and hash can be. In fact, the potency of any THC drug is increased (that is, increased in feeling) by eating rather than smoking, any pill should be eaten (as opposed to shooting).

It makes little difference to the body whether the drug is eaten alone or in combination with other foods (which is a good idea with some not-so-pleasant organic drugs such as mescaline), except for the fact that it will be digested faster if the stomach has more to work on than a small pill.

Coke and heroin especially lose great amounts of their potency when digested.

SMOKING

Many drugs can be smoked: Heroin, DMT, grass, hash, opium, etc. Some drugs such as LSD are ineffective when smoked as heat tends to break them down chemically before they enter the user's system.

Any THC-involved product is normally smoked. Hash may be added to tobacco or to grass or even smoked in a small pipe by it-

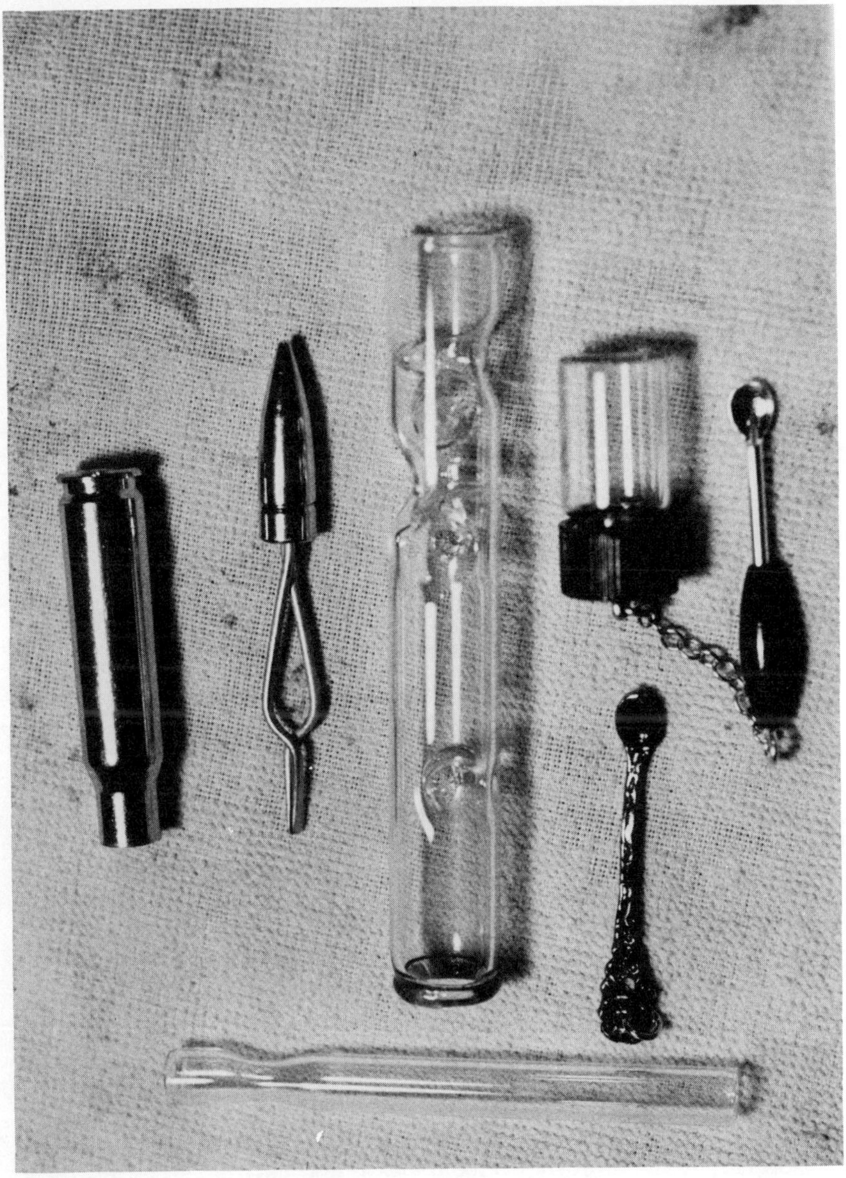

COMMON DOPE INSTRUMENTS OF DESTRUCTION: Roach clip, glass, tube for snorting coke, coke spoon and spoon and storage bottle combination and even a small glass carburetor.

self. Grass is usually smoked in a rolled-up cigarette paper or in a water pipe or carburetor.

The water pipe exposes the smoke to a body of cool water or wine which slightly filters the smoke, cools it, and in the case of wine, makes it a bit less harsh, before entering your lungs.

A carburetor is a device for mixing the smoke with the correct quantity of air and cooling it before inhaling. A good carburetor will increase the high somewhat, but no device will turn bad dope into good dope.

DMT and DET are smoked in VERY minute quantities like 30 milligrams. Organic DMT is usually placed on a small quantity of parsley in an open dish. The DMT is ignited and the first cloud or two of smoke inhaled deeply into the lungs.

SHOOTING

Many drugs can be shot or injected, but, as it gives the most concentrated stone in the shortest period of time, this is also the most risky form of ingestion.

An outfit or "fit" is preferred by most needle freaks. This consists of a nose dropper with a rubber bulb from a baby's pacifier on the large end and a hypodermic needle on the other. This arrangement gives the user a much more controlled situation than a hypodermic syringe does.

The drug is dissolved in water (some drugs such as speed dissolve automatically, others such as street level heroin must be "cooked," usually in a bottle cap or spoon, to dissolve.) Normally, the quicker and cleaner a drug dissolves, the purer it can be expected to be. Then it is drawn up into the fit by suction from the rubber bulb.

Most drugs are shot directly into a vein, although some of the more potent drugs such as heroin, can be inter-muscularly injected or "popped," shot directly under the skin and allowed to enter the system at a slower rate.

Mainline injections are meant to be made into a vein, NOT AN ARTERY! Arteries deliver blood from the heart to individual tissue masses such as the hands, feet, etc., whereas veins deliver the blood FROM tissues into the heart.

When drugs are injected into an artery, high concentrations of the drug are immediately shoved into a relatively small area (such as a hand) and has the potential of severe damage to that area.

When a drug such as a red is mainlined into an artery, the highly alkaline salts rush to the tissue mass and can cause severe damage including gangrene.

When the same drug is shot into a vein, it is carried to the heart and divided among all the arteries of the body avoiding the centralized damage syndrome.

Common symptoms of a miss-shot (into an artery) are immediate pain, swelling, a feeling of the area being on fire (where the drug is doing the damage). Abscesses, blisters, and visible tissue poisoning can also result right after the injection.

The "advantage" to shooting is a more direct high, usually a "flash" or rush (an extreme reaction as the drug reaches the nerve centers) happens first with the stone following directly afterwards. This quick reaction makes impatient users more likely to shoot drugs which are as effective even when swallowed, such as psychedelics.

Once the drug is in the fit, the needle is inserted into a vein. Usually the user will tie a tight band such as a belt or surgical rubber tube around the body above the vein to be used to make the vein stand out clearer. As the needle enters a vein, the user relaxes the pressure on the bulb and a stream of bright red blood, or a "flag" is drawn up into the tube. This flag reaction indicates the user has the needle correctly inserted into a vein. The rubber bulb is then fully depressed and the drug is injected into the body.

Heroin is almost always shot, especially by more experienced addicts. Coke can be, and in fact, gives a much higher "rush" when this is done but the total reaction dissipates quicker than when it is sniffed. Most all the psychedelics can be shot, and people have even attempted to shoot liquid soups of marijuana. In fact, a couple of people have died from this stupidity.

Shooting is risky — no way around it. Any impurities or other bad things are put directly into the bloodstream and into the brain without any bodily filtering. Abscesses can form from dirty needles. Veins harden up with use, and heavy addicts must constantly search for virgin veins to hit in. These hardened veins leave dark purple and black scars which just can't be explained away to curious onlookers or policemen. Even light shooting leaves "tracks" or needle marks which are always a bummer when stopped by the police or questioned by relatives.

Hepatitis is a very real danger to anyone who uses or allows another to use common needles.

Some drugs are rejected by the body when shoved on it in such great concentrations and form long, red, blood poisoning marks or sores. Some drugs are fine but are cut with other substances which the body cannot cope with directly into the bloodstream.

Needle freaks are also subject to a strange malady known as needle happiness. This is a reaction which would appear to be wholly psychological in any medical sense, but can and does approach physiological proportions in seasoned users.

A freak who is needle happy digs the drugs, sure, but he digs the needle as much or more. This results in the freak shooting a drug in several small injections to experience the needle rush over and over, or shooting and sucking the drug mixed with blood, back into the needle and shooting again. Strong needle lovers get to the point where the needle is everything. They will shoot Kool-aid, sugar water, or coffee just for the slight chemical rush and the needle.

Real hard-nosed needle freaks or heavy addicts get to the point where finding a virgin place to shoot is a major operation. Some resort to crotch shooting or under-the-tongue shots.

If you just gotta shoot there are several things you can do to minimize the inevitable damage:

NEVER share your needle or use anyone else's.

ALWAYS boil your whole fit for at least 15 minutes before using.

NEVER shoot anything which you are not sure of or are not sure of the purity.

NEVER shoot pills, or if you choose to ignore this advice, ALWAYS let the pills soak for at least one hour in a quantity of water and ONLY shoot the clear solution, NEVER THE POWDER! Some commercial filling agents can cause blindness when injected directly into the bloodstream.

SNIFFING

Some drugs can be inhaled up through the nose and absorbed by the small blood vessels located in the mucous membranes. This gets the drug into the bloodstream near the brain with little loss.

Generally the more "body" drugs can be successfully sniffed and not the mind drugs.

Cocaine is almost always sniffed. Heroin can be and speed can be but most psychedelics will not sniff well.

Sniffing on a regular basis is hard on the delicate membranes in the nose. (Sigmund Freud, a confirmed coke addict, had to have three separate nose operations due to his incessant sniffing.) If you are going to sniff, first make sure the drug is chopped as fine as it will go. If necessary, crush with a heavy object or mortar and pestle into a fine powder. NEVER sniff rocks! Make sure the nose is clear. Nose drops are good for this purpose.

Place the drug on a clean surface, arrange it into two thin "streaks." Use a small tube designed for this purpose or roll up a dollar bill very tightly and place one end in one nostril. Place the other end on the beginning of the streak, close the other nostril and inhale hard and suddenly, moving the tube down the streak until all the drug is in your nose. Close the nostril with your finger and sniff hard. Suddenly release the finger while continuing to sniff. Repeat the process with the other nostril.

Now take some pure (or better yet, distilled) water and snuff it up both nostrils several times. This will help wash the raw membrane and will free any little particles that have stuck to the nostril.

ETC.

There are a couple of less popular but still existing methods for taking drugs. Many organic drugs such as grass, hash, yage, yohimbe, etc., can be boiled into a tea and drunk or cooked with foods and eaten.

Some people place dissolvable drugs under the tongue rather than swallowing them. A mass of small veins runs very close to the surface here, and it is reported one can get the drug into the bloodstream in a shorter period of time than with swallowing. Of course, this is not recommended with any drug that tastes bad (speed, coke, weird acid tabs, etc.), as the horror will stay in your mouth for some time.

Some native tribes in South America and Africa have a novel method of consuming organic drugs such as yage. They place a finger full up the anal passage and literally sit on their high. In these countries the term "stick it up your ass" is not always regarded as an insult.

THE MAKE-YOUR-OWN-IMPLEMENT PAGE

A great way to get personal satisfaction, as well as impress the hell out of your noncreative, dope-smoking friends, is to design and create your own paraphernalia. With a trifle bit of creativity and common household throwaways, even you can work wonders.

First, assemble a typical household pile of throwaways, a few tools that suit your fancy, and a large joint. Now, light up the joint and pick up the first tool. Take another toke on the joint, pick up the first discard, take another toke on the joint. . .

Alligator clips are one of the handiest items for the do-it-yourselfer. An electrical alligator clip and a bit of glue (or tape) can transform almost any inanimate object into a roach clip. A patent pending, superexpandable roach clip can be easily constructed by attaching aforementioned alligator clip to any spare rabbit ear antenna. In this fashion, one person can regulate the intake of a whole crowd.

Probably, the greatest roach clip around is a doctor's hemostat. This little goody can often be found in surplus stores, along with a whole slough of other handy gadgets for the implement maker.

Hash pipes can be carved from general artist materials; from deer antlers, molded and baked out of clay; or even totally constructed from mini-pipes and joints available at any plumbers' supply house to create a sort of art-nouveau look in toke pipes.

Chillums can be ceramically constructed in a home oven. Stash boxes can be fashioned from jewelry and makeup cases, dime store rings can be turned into poison rings, and even the bones of dead animals and/or friends can be hollowed out for pipes or chillums.

The newest addition to the paraphernalia tree of life is the concert pipe; a small combination carburetor and device for holding much of the smoke/smell in. A crude, but nonetheless, effective, facsimile can be put together with a small plastic aspirin bottle, which has a tapered mouthpiece, a wire for joint holding and a small hole (for the necessary dosages of O_2) in the cover, added to its basic configuration.

Of course, the ultimate home brew trip aid is the ancient device known as the air enhancer chamber. This modern version is an updated application of the one employed in the rites performed when a pharoah died.

First: Close all windows in your house or apartment. Now, hang plastic (dry cleaners bags glued together will suffice in a pinch) all over the walls and doorway of one room. Place a quantity (about two pounds is generally used) of marijuana in the center of the room directly over a can of sterno. Now, light the sterno, run around the room in concentric circles until you are exhausted and breathing heavily. Hyperventilation is good at this point.

This produces a definite spiritual trip, from which, users occasionally never recover.

OF COURSE, YOU CAN GET CARRIED AWAY WITH IMPRESSING YOUR FRIENDS. . .

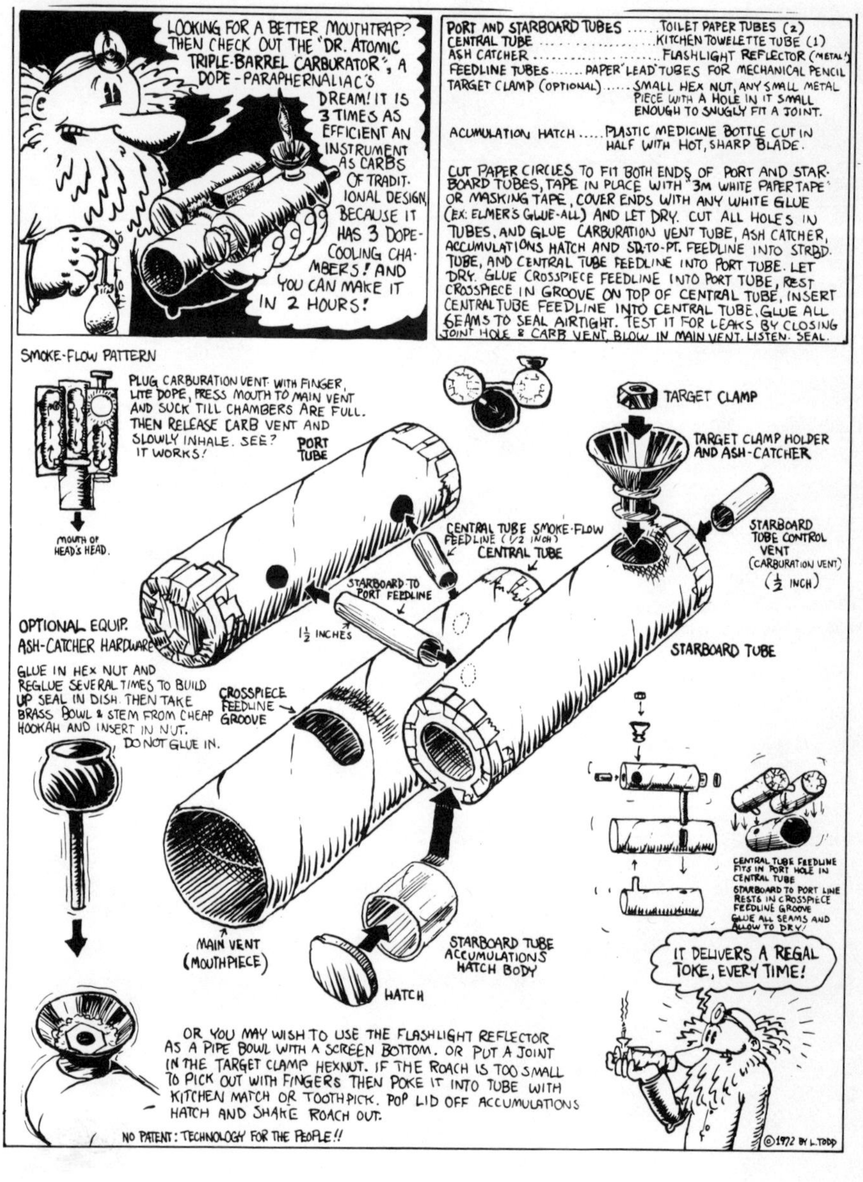

Dr. Atomic's Triple Barrel Carburetor, it really works! Reprinted by permission.

COST OF LIVING

The dope market is a perfect mini-economic system model. The prices, quantities, and even terminology have responded to the laws of supply and demand in a way obvious even to those of us on the shitty end of the economic stick (consumers).

Back in the merry days of Haight and Hippies, LSD was the magic drug. The processes were fairly secret and the drug's popularity was migrating eastward via the college campus route. The average acid tab sold for $2.50 to $5.00, with some economic tourist holdouts, such as Florida, getting as much as $10.00 a hit. . .

Now, with the slackening in demand, and the organic "simpler" processes, as well as the general abundance of freaked-out chemists, the average tab gets $0.50 – $0.75 with the cream of the crop (such as Clear Light) commanding a street high of $2.00 – $3.00.

Magic mairjuana, on the other hand, having become the socially "in" drug for the cocktail set, which has created a high demand, has fallen prey to price and quantity manipulators.

In the late '60's, a key (a real kilo, mind you) of top Mexican weed could easily be had for $160, or less, depending on your standing in the pipeline pecking order. The price started to rise until it became prohibitive to talk about keys, so people began selling "bricks," some undefined, vague chunk of marijuana usually weighing in at 1½ – 2 pounds. This brick could be sold for a price which seemed reasonable to people who were used to buying $200 keys, and it seemed so much better to buy a $200 brick than a $300 key. . .

As the prices inflated further, the brick shrank and shrank (after all, when there was no real standard size, how could you yell "cheat". . .). At some point, the brick gave way to another Madison Avenue type price reduction — it became a pound.

Now, one easily pays $100 a pound for even mediocre weed and up to/through $400 a pound for top of the line, made-in-the-middle-of-the-week superweed.

These same evil economic forces are hard at work in the harder drugs where the price of heroin and coke have jumped wildly upward while the strength and the size of the "spoons" have gone spiraling downward.

The moral of all this is: like unpopular drugs; abstain; or use only pre-

scription/over-the-counter drugs which are already wildly overpriced and unlikely to rise much more.

Of course, one must develop a certain taste for Romilar every night, but it could certainly be no worse than drinking cheap scotch, right?

FUTURE TRIPS AND MISCELLANEOUS RAMBLINGS

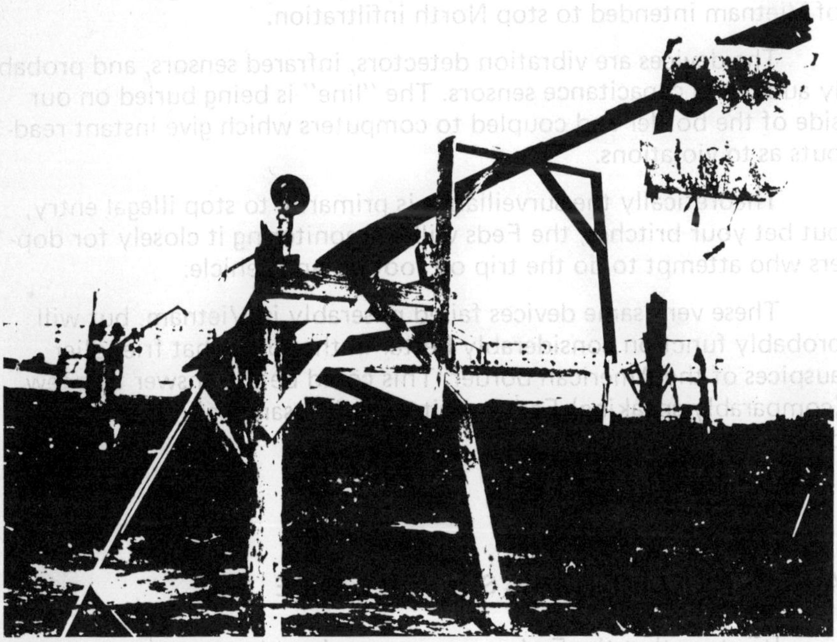

FUTURE TRIPS AND MISCELLANEOUS RAMBLINGS

The United States government is currently in the process of electronically "fencing in" the Mexican-American border. About 100 miles is known to be operational as of this writing, with the entire border to be bugged by the mid-seventies.

The devices used are government surplus from the "great Vietnam conflict," where they were employed in the "McNamara Line," an invisible line of electronic security devices stretching across parts of Vietnam intended to stop North infiltration.

The devices are vibration detectors, infrared sensors, and probably audio and capacitance sensors. The "line" is being buried on our side of the border and coupled to computers which give instant readouts as to violations.

Theoretically the surveillance is primarily to stop illegal entry, but bet your britches, the Feds will be monitoring it closely for dopers who attempt to do the trip on foot or land vehicle.

These very same devices failed miserably in Vietnam, but will probably function considerably better in the somewhat friendlier auspices of the American border. This could be the answer to a few (comparably speaking) Feds monitoring thousands of miles of border.

Watch for it.

AIRBORNE ELECTRONIC SURVEILLANCE

It is true that the Feds can spot any sizeable quantity of marijuana from the air by using a device which identifies the plant's "electronic fingerprints" as registered on an infrared sensor.

It is also true that America the beautiful has satellites orbiting, right this second, as you read this very paragraph, which can also identify certain flora and fauna by its infrared traces and does so on a daily basis. However, this satellite monitoring is used only (so far, that is) on large fields of marijuana and poppies. This sort of surveillance gives the U.S. government the political clout it needs to make the other governments crack down on such activity within its borders.

The airplane brand of electronic surveillance can identify much smaller patches of devil weed than its orbiting counterpart and must be assumed to be in effect in hot areas (such as the Midwest) to spot natural grass as well as pick out fields of corn which are impregnated with cultivated marijuana.

SCHIZOID FUN

The human body manufactures, in minute quantities, a drug known as adrenochrome. This drug is thought to be related to the functioning of the adrenal glands and very much resembles (in chemical makeup) several psychotropic drugs, notably mescaline.

This drug is found in larger quantities in the blood of people afflicted with schizophrenia. It was once rumored that Salvador Dali had an extremely large concentration of adrenochrome in his vital fluids. . .

At any rate, drug freaks, always looking for a new high, can probably be expected to begin shooting up the blood of schizo friends. This would be especially probably in dry times, when other, more conventional drugs are hard to get. This procedure would, of course, open up new fields of endeavor for schizophrenics and crooked psychiatrists, and possibly allow the schizophrenic to make a viable contribution to society.

FUTURE STONES

The state of the art in psychedelic chemistry is a long way from being reached. Numerous chemists are starting to scratch the surface in drug preparation. A couple of good combined works have been recently published in this field which show some of the possibilities.

There are still hundreds of natural-occurring psychoactive drugs scattered around the world, some of which are in use by various "natives," and some of which are still waiting to be eaten, smoked, snuffed, or stuffed (see imbibing section).

At the same time, there are literally hundreds or maybe thousands of analogs and derivatives of now illegal psychedelics which have never been outlawed, not because of any less "danger" or potency, but because they are not manufactured in any quantity.

Examples of the latter are 5-MEO-DMT: the possible isomers, analogs, and homologs of THC such as delta 3's (the delta sign indicates the position of the double bond in THC synthesis); and the analogs of the common (er) delta 1 and delta 6 synthesis; or the possible DET, DPT, other DMT analogs and isomers; as well as syntheses of yet legal, organically derived drugs. Of course, as each of these achieves any notoriety they will, no doubt, be outlawed by those people who are appointed to help us govern ourselves, but then the wise chemist moves on to the next drug.

Anyone who has the experience and nerve to attempt these experimental drugs should be advised to stay on top of the laws as they are passed.

We will also probably begin to see a more plentiful supply of cocaine as it is very possible to synthesize (although the process is quite difficult), but the increasing popularity and price of coke will probably soon lead people into attempting the manufacture.

It is very possible that we will soon see a couple of different varieties of "grass" as the popular hops/marijuana cross becomes available. (Of course, we will also see the authorities watching hops growing a bit more also.) We may well soon see the first chemically produced THC or THC analog added to alfalfa for a "super weed," BUT be sure – test it. Either of these "super grasses" could be produced for less money than the imported variety.

It is also interesting to note that the popularity of alcohol, especially among the Pepsi generation, is very definitely on the upswing.

Who knows? Maybe we'll all become AA freaks.

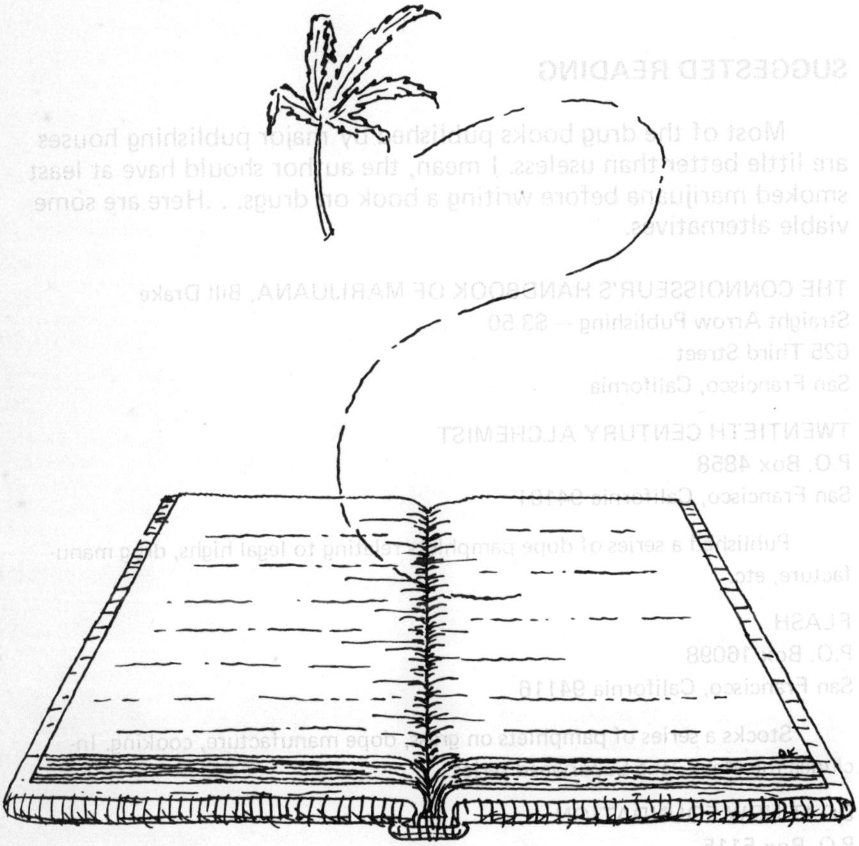

recommended reading

SUGGESTED READING

Most of the drug books published by major publishing houses are little better than useless. I mean, the author should have at least smoked marijuana before writing a book on drugs. . .Here are some viable alternatives.

THE CONNOISSEUR'S HANDBOOK OF MARIJUANA, Bill Drake
Straight Arrow Publishing — $3.50
625 Third Street
San Francisco, California

TWENTIETH CENTURY ALCHEMIST
P.O. Box 4858
San Francisco, California 94101

Published a series of dope pamphlets relating to legal highs, drug manufacture, etc.

FLASH
P.O. Box 16098
San Francisco, California 94116

Stocks a series of pamphlets on grass, dope manufacture, cooking. Includes the Mary Jane Superweed series.

DO IT NOW FOUNDATION
P.O. Box 5115
Phoenix, Arizona 85010

A foundation for the study and unbiased reporting of dope and dope-related trips. Puts together the dope news in the L.A. Free Press and operates a street clinic and testing facility in L.A. Many pamphlets, records, and films. Especially good for educators and groups.

THE STUDENT ASSOCIATION FOR THE STUDY OF HALLUCINOGENS, INC.
638 Pleasant Street
Beloit, Wisconsin 53511

A coordinating agency for the study of drugs. They publish a series of newsletters ($5.00 per year) and a monthly journal (Grassroots, $95.00 per year) which scans over 600 other journals and reports every month and does a capsule summary on the available data. Grassroots also gives a bimonthly bibliography on current drug literature and publishes a yearly directory listing 2,000 drug organizations across the country.

HAIGHT ASHBURY MEDICAL CLINIC
558 Clayton Street
San Francisco, California 94117

Publishes a series of books dealing with drugs and drug experiences, including Psychedelic Drugs and Religion, Psychedelic Drugs and the Law, etc.

PSYCHEDELIC CHEMISTRY
Rip Off Press – $4.95
1250 Seventeenth Street
San Francisco, California

This book is the most authoritative manual on drug chemistry ever assembled. Exact, very exact, directions for the concoction of practically every drug known to man or beast, BUT, this is written in terms that an advanced organic chemist could deal with, and no one else. IT is NOT a do-it-yourself-in-the-kitchen-and-become-rich manual. The book is put together by Michael Valentine Smith (shades of Stranger in a Strange Land) who, is in reality, a university professor at a western university.

Much of the book was done with the help of the university's computer. . .

SCHOOL OF PHARMACY
University of the Pacific
Stockton, California 95024

A series of bulletins about drugs and street dealing put together by several professors of pharmacology.

PHYSICIANS DESK REFERENCE

THE book on pharmaceutical drugs. Lists every commercial drug, along with pictures, identifying marks and dosages.

ORBA Information, Ltd.
418 Saint Sulpice Street
Montreal 125, CANADA

ORBA is a weekly news service which reads some 285 publications searching for news of drugs, alcohol and tobacco doings.

The weekly report summarizes any findings and lists the original source if you care to get the whole article. All of this is done on an international scale for the sum of $60 a year (includes airmail postage with each subscription).